Love, Hope, Lyme

What Family Members, Partners, and Friends Who Love a Chronic Lyme Survivor Need to Know

Praise for *Love, Hope, Lyme*

"Fred Diamond has done a great service to the Lyme community by writing Love, Hope, Lyme. People with chronic illness need support—often physical support, but always emotional support, and Fred details the ways wives, husbands, and friends can help those who have chronic Lyme disease. I agree with Fred that hope is key, and when Lyme patients themselves feel hopeless, loved ones can hold it for them with compassion and love. Most people with chronic Lyme get better, and sometimes they need to be reminded of that on a daily basis. Fred gives an excellent overview of how you can help a loved one with this illness."
—*Daniel A. Kinderlehrer MD, author of* Recovery from Lyme Disease: The Integrative Medicine Guide to Diagnosing and Treating Tick-Borne Illness

"Finally, a resource for our spouses. If this book existed a decade ago, my relationship would have survived my recovery journey."
—*Yessi Young, author of* It's Not Just Lyme: Understanding the Metabolism's Role in Fighting Chronic Infections

"This is the book everyone who loves a person with Lyme disease or any chronic illness needs to read. What a beautiful guide to navigating the journey in a better and more supportive way as a partner."
—*Amy B. Scher, author of* This Is How I Save My Life: Searching the World for a Cure: A Lyme Disease Memoir

"*Love, Hope, Lyme* is as an excellent resource for patients and their families who are beginning the long and difficult Lyme journey. It is filled with excellent information, and it would be great if it could reach as many Lyme-suffering families as possible."
—*Dr. Neil Nathan, author of* Toxic: Heal Your Body from Mold Toxicity, Lyme Disease, Multiple Chemical Sensitivities, and Chronic Environmental Illness

"Fred Diamond captures the mystery, frustration, and agony of watching a loved one who is suffering from Lyme Borreliosis Complex (LBC) in his book,

Love, Hope, Lyme. This primary focus of the book is to counsel others in a similar support situation where challenges abound and accurate answers are seldom found. This is a valuable work for the primary support person dealing with a complex, often devastating and misunderstood chronic illness. I applaud Fred for his perseverance in learning about LBC as well as his compassion and love for his partner. I have certainly seen a high percentage of marriages/relationships shattered due to this health dynamic; hopefully, Fred's insight and generosity in sharing what he has discovered will keep more couples together in the future."

—*Joseph G. Jemsek, MD, FACP*

"Fred Diamond's must-read book has provided us with an amazing overview of Lyme disease through the eyes of a loving partner. By doing his homework, Fred opens a unique window into the pain, questions, and consequences this truly insidious disease can wield on those stricken, and on the devoted family members who support them."

—*Zev Halpern, Licensed Relationship Counselor/Coach*

"It is difficult for partners, family, and friends to understand the hardship of an invisible illness like Lyme disease. *Love, Hope, Lyme* is an excellent guide on how to support a loved one with chronic Lyme disease. I highly recommend it!"

—*Todd A. Maderis, ND, Medical Director, Marin Natural Medicine Clinic*

Love, Hope, Lyme

What Family Members, Partners, and Friends Who Love a Chronic Lyme Survivor Need to Know

BY FRED DIAMOND

Copyright © 2022 Fred Diamond

Cover Art copyright © 2022 Tim Ford

ISBN: 979-8-9862077-1-1

Published by Fred Diamond

Edited by Wendi M. Lindenmuth

All rights reserved.

No part of this publication may be reproduced, stored in a retrieval system, or transmitted in any form or by any means, electronic, mechanical, photocopying, recording, scanning, or otherwise, without prior written consent by the author.

The fact that an individual, organization, or website is referred to in this work as a citation and/or potential source of further information does not mean that the author endorses the information the individual, organization, or website may provide or recommendations they/it may make. Further, readers should be aware that websites listed in this work may have changed or disappeared between when this work was written and when it is read. People mentioned in Chapter 6 have given their approval to be included in this book.

The Lyme symptoms described in this book are not ascribed to any specific person, living or dead, except where duly noted. They are all included in this book based on independent research on the topic by the author. Any similarity of events, incidents, or occurrences, or any resemblance, similarity or attribution to a specific person or persons, is purely coincidental.

Dedication

*To Lyme disease survivors around the globe.
Have hope. Be loved.*

Table of Contents

Disclaimer	11
Letter to the Reader	13
Introduction	17
Prologue	21
Chapter One: My Journey to Understand Lyme Disease Begins	23
Chapter Two: What You Need to Know about Lyme Disease	31
Chapter Three: The Challenges of Understanding Lyme Disease	41
Chapter Four: More Lyme Disease Terms to Know	45
Chapter Five: Neurological Concerns	51
Chapter Six: Stories of Lyme Survivors and How You Can Make a Difference	55
Chapter Seven: The Little Things You Can Do to Make Everyone's Life Easier	65
Chapter Eight: Covering Family Activities	69
Chapter Nine: Step Up Your Game Because She Deserves It	73
Chapter Ten: Facebook Helped Me—It Might Help You	79
Chapter Eleven: Being Gluten-Free Before It Was Cool	87
Chapter Twelve: The Six Stages of Healing	91
Chapter Thirteen: Politics, Expense, Insurance	97
Chapter Fourteen: Becoming Your Own Health Care Advocate	105
Chapter Fifteen: What Lyme Survivors Ask Each Other	113
Chapter Sixteen: Love, Cherish, and Laugh	117
Chapter Seventeen: Final Thoughts	119
References	121
Appendix A: Fifteen Books About Lyme I Recommend	125
Acknowledgments	131
About the Author	133
Epilogue	135

Disclaimer

This book does not provide medical advice. All information obtained from this book is to be taken solely as advisory in nature. The author does not dispense medical or other professional advice or prescribe the use of any technique as a form of diagnosis or treatment for any physical, emotional, or mental conditions. The content and information regarding Lyme disease are for informational purposes only. No material in this book is intended to be a substitute for professional medical advice, diagnosis, or treatment. Always seek the advice of a qualified health care provider with any questions you may have regarding a medical condition or treatment and before undertaking any new health care regimen, and never disregard professional medical advice or delay seeking it because of something that you read in this book.

The author's intent is only to offer information of an anecdotal and general nature that may be part of your loved one's quest for emotional, mental, physical, and spiritual well-being. The author assumes no responsibility for the direct or indirect consequences, losses, incidental, special, or consequential damages arising out of or in any way connected with the use of any of the content of this book. The author shall not be held personally, legally, or financially liable for any action taken based upon suggestions found in this book.

The reader should consult their medical, health, or other professional before using any of the book's suggestions or drawing inferences from it. The reader acknowledges that they assume full responsibility for all the information gleaned from reading this book and assume any liability for the consequences of applying such information.

Letter to the Reader

Thank you for reading *Love, Hope, Lyme*.

If your partner, child, parent, or friend is a chronic Lyme disease survivor, this book should help you understand the struggles and challenges of Lyme disease and how to support someone you love.

You should know a few things.

I don't have Lyme disease, nor have I ever have had it. I also do not have the credentials to offer medical advice. I'm a history major with an MBA.

I don't know what it feels like to suffer from a disease that impacts every part of your body and might change your life forever.

I don't know what it feels like to be alone with no support.

At one time, all I thought you needed to do to support a Lyme disease survivor was to maintain a stress-free environment for them and know where to find the best gluten-free pizza.

When I decided to learn more about Lyme disease, I realized I had a lot to learn. And here are some things I learned along the way.

I found out that there was not a lot of guidance for the partners and families of chronic Lyme survivors who want to know how to support the person they care about to get their health back.

There are some excellent books on treating the disease and some exceptional first-person testimonials about what life with this mysterious disease could be like, and I've read most of them. But there is no short, straightforward guide for partners and family members to understand what their loved one is going through.

So here it is.

According to the Centers for Disease Control (CDC) website (more about the CDC later), I discovered that nearly 500,000 people are newly infected by Lyme disease and other tick-borne diseases every year in the United States alone. It's an epidemic.

I discovered that other complications from ticks called coinfections can wear down a person's immune system.

Some of these coinfections are parasites that can get triggered during stress and trauma. The coinfections can be just as harmful as Lyme disease.

I was dumbfounded by the lack of health care providers who were Lyme literate and could provide effective treatment.

I did not know that there were political issues with Lyme disease.

I was appalled to learn that some official bodies did not acknowledge that *chronic Lyme* existed, even in cases where their own testing criteria might still show an active infection after the standard thirty days of antibiotic treatment.

I did not know that insurance companies rarely covered Lyme treatment past thirty days. Insurance companies will, for the most part, cover medicine unless it is injected via intravenous (IV) or intramuscular (IM). Some drugs will be covered, but they typically do not cover Lyme-literate medical doctor (LLMD) visits or specialty testing.

Participating in multiple Lyme disease online support groups, I saw that many marriages and relationships ended due to the stress, lack of support, and the partner's lack of understanding about the disease and its effects. In addition, I was disheartened to hear that family members and close friends do not always believe their loved ones suffer from this disease.

I also learned about the extremes to which people have gone to treat the symptoms. Medicine commonly known to treat parasites in horses, ingredients found in kitty litter, and machines that fought the infections by zeroing in on radio frequencies were widely used.

I was unaware that people might have gone decades without knowing they even had Lyme disease, yet they endured constant pain and fatigue.

I did not know the challenges with healing.

So I searched "Lyme disease and partner" on the internet and then purchased dozens of books on Lyme disease, women's illness, and anxiety to educate myself further. I read them all and contacted many of the authors.

I reached out to everyone who ever uttered "Lyme" to me in the past ten years.

I sought out every Lyme organization I could find.

I asked Lyme survivors questions and befriended many of them.

I listened to Lyme podcasts.

Although I was consuming all this information, the most important thing I was looking for and could not find was a book on how to support your partner or family member who has Lyme disease.

What I discovered is there wasn't one.

So I wrote one.

I intend for this book to be read by partners, family, and friends who need and want to learn more about supporting a loved one with chronic Lyme disease.

Thank you for reading this book. I hope it helps you to better understand this illness and to be a source of comfort and strength to those suffering from it.

Fred Diamond
Vienna, Virginia
June 2022

Introduction
By Dr. Richard Horowitz

When I was first asked to write the introduction for Fred Diamond's new book *Love, Hope, Lyme*, I thought it was going to be another self-healing book on the topic. I was pleasantly surprised to find that the tone and message of the book was an essential topic, considering the depth and breadth of the Lyme epidemic, with a message that was not adequately covered by other books on the subject.

Many of us live with loved ones who are chronic disease survivors. That has also been the story of my life. Before I met my beloved wife, Lee, who suffered with Lyme-Multiple Systemic Infectious Disease Syndrome (MSIDS), one of my prior relationships was destroyed by Lyme disease. No matter how well-intentioned I was, even as a Lyme-literate provider, I could not find a healing path in that relationship. The challenges of loving someone and caring for them on a regular basis, putting someone else's needs above your own, can easily destroy a relationship if you and/or your partner have not been adequately trained in the art of loving and caring for yourself and others, and/or if the foundation of that relationship is not rock solid.

This book provides a guidepost for those living with loved ones with a chronic illness and explains how we can approach our loved ones with sensitivity, care, compassion, and understanding. This also happens to be a common-sense and wise approach as to how we can best live our own lives too. Love is wanting others to be happy, and compassion is wanting other people to be free from suffering. We all want that for ourselves and for those we deeply care about. The stories of suffering and healing in this book are stories we all experience, will experience, or have experienced during our lifetime. Learning how to be sensitive to our own and others' needs are essential tools we must have in our relationship toolbox if we expect to have happy and fulfilling lives.

I am fortunate to have now married a woman with a big heart and joyful disposition, even when she was ill. Not everyone has that gift handed to them. I've learned a lot from my wife, Lee. I had to learn to never give up in the name of love, and to keep pressing onward, making sure I was always doing my best. Love would have me do no less. My wife is now well after diagnosing and treating all of the abnormalities on the sixteen-point MSIDS map, described in my last book, *How Can I Get Better? An Action Plan for Treating Resistant Lyme and Chronic Disease*. It was not an easy journey, yet it was a worthwhile one. Our relationship is stronger because of it.

These sixteen MSIDS variables, which I have found to be present in the majority of the 13,000 chronic Lyme disease patients I have treated over the past thirty-plus years, are from my perspective the medical solutions most people are looking for. Especially effective are the newer treatments with persister drugs, like dapsone combination therapy, which I have published information about in the medical literature during the past several years. I now have many patients going into long-term remission with only a few months of oral antibiotics. Yet, even with the best of treatments for properly addressing Lyme, Babesia, Bartonella, adrenal dysfunction, Postural Orthostatic Tachycardia Syndrome (POTS), food allergies and sensitivities, mast cell activation, mold and heavy metals, sleep disorders, hormonal and mitochondrial dysfunction, and other abnormalities on the MSIDS map, one of the most difficult variables to transform is the psychological aspect of the illness, and how it affects afflicted individuals and those around them.

Healing in its greatest form must include healing of the body, mind, emotions, and spirit. Fred's book puts front and center the big issues most Lyme patients will have to deal with, but more importantly, it discusses the ephemeral and transcendental virtue of love, and how that ultimately can bring some of the greatest healing. With love comes hope, and when love and hope are mixed with the right medical knowledge, healing can and does happen.

Whether you are living with a loved one compromised by a chronic illness, or whether you yourself suffer with Lyme and associated infections, the messages of this book will always stand the test of time. Because love is eternal and brings forth hope and healing. I wish you blessings on your healing journey. Let the messages in this book be an inspiration for you and your loved one to go forth and live your lives with love, hope, compassion, and a sense of purpose.

The difficult lessons that we learn in this life are often our greatest teachers, pushing us forward evolutionarily even when we go kicking and screaming. Let this book be a rudder for your ship during difficult times. If you persist and never give up in the name of love, hope will find a strong foundation, and your life, and the life of your loved one, will be all the more enriched because of it.

—Dr. Richard Horowitz, May 8, Mother's Day, 2022

Prologue

The Dalai Lama once said, "I love everything in the world . . . except for ticks."

This book was written as if your loved one is a woman. It is not my intent, however, to be gender-specific nor exclusive. As the Lyme disease epidemic grows, everyone and anyone can be inflicted with Lyme disease and other tick-borne illnesses.

Relationships evolve, morph, and shift. The status of a relationship, whether active or in the past, such as this one, isn't important in the context of this book. Understanding the epidemic that is Lyme disease, and how to support someone you love who has it, is what matters.

CHAPTER ONE
My Journey to Understand Lyme Disease Begins

In the summer of 2021, I decided to learn more about my partner's chronic Lyme disease.

I wondered if I really knew how it affected her.

That summer, I began a journey to understand what chronic Lyme survivors went through on a day-by-day basis.

- When did their symptoms start?
- How did their symptoms show up every day?
- Are they the same symptoms every day or different?
- What did the disease do to their bodies and minds?
- What caused the disease to do what it did?
- Was it curable?

I realized that my understanding of the disease was quite basic, so I took it upon myself to learn as much as possible to be more helpful. Along the way, I learned a lot about the community of Lyme survivors and how difficult it could be to get support from family, friends, and even the medical establishment.

For example, on the social media groups I joined, I frequently saw posts from Lyme survivors wishing that partners and other family members would learn more to understand this disease.

Chronic Lyme disease is a hidden epidemic that is hard to understand unless you have it. Most people do not understand this mysterious disease. If anything, they may know that it is most likely caused by a tick bite and may cause fatigue, but little more. As a result, many survivors feel alone and isolated. There is limited and conflicting knowledge about treating the disease, so the struggle to get healthy is a constant battle. As a partner, family member, or friend, you can only empathize, support, and show interest and care.

Life has changed. Your loved one's way of functioning may be different than before. She may move a little slower, think a little longer, and become tired more quickly. This may be temporary, or not exhibit itself for years.

For her to function at her best, lifestyle adjustments may be needed. In speaking with many Lyme survivors, I learned an overabundance of patience goes a long way in helping your partner feel valued and less stressed.

I saw a Lyme survivor post the following poem on Facebook that reflects this:

> *I miss me*
> *The old me*
> *The smiling me*
> *The laughing me*
> *The gone me*

Unfortunately, the Lyme world is full of broken relationships, pain, and suffering.

But there is always hope. Amazing lives can be had, and you'll learn about some people who continue to do great things later in this book.

I hope that this book will help you establish a better relationship with your loved one living with Lyme disease. The possibilities to continue growing a powerful relationship are endless.

Not everyone with Lyme disease experiences the same exact symptoms. Many feel well for extended periods of time, while others never do.

Many get to the point where they can have spectacular and fulfilling lives. In chapter six, I'll introduce you to some Lyme survivors who found their life's mission while treating the disease. It is important to know what type of symptoms are common for chronic Lyme survivors, so you have an idea of what to expect.

Many Lyme survivors, I've found, do not want to be treated like puppy dogs, but they do want those who love them to know what they go through.

Here are some symptoms Lyme survivors may experience. All these stages may overlap, and neuropsychiatric symptoms can be present even early on.

Early-Stage Lyme disease
- Chills
- Fatigue
- Fever
- Headache
- Joint pain and swelling
- Muscle pain
- Rash
- Swelling of the lymph nodes

Late-Stage Lyme disease

Late-stage Lyme disease symptoms may appear days to months after the initial tick bite and may include but are not limited to:

- Additional rashes in new places on the body
- Arthritis or joint pain and swelling, especially of large joints (such as the knee)
- Dizziness or shortness of breath
- Facial palsy, also known as Bell's palsy—paralysis of one side of the face
- Heart palpitations or arrhythmia
- Inflammation of the brain or spinal cord
- Intermittent tendon, muscle, joint, nerve, or bone pain
- Severe headaches and neck stiffness
- Shooting pains, numbness, or tingling in the hands or feet
- Anxiety and paranoia
- Chronic inflammation
- Dizziness and shortness of breath
- Dysphonia (vocal cord damage)
- Fibromyalgia
- Hallucinations

- Hearing sensitivity
- Heart palpitations and irregular heartbeat
- Intermittent fevers, chills, and sweats
- Joint pain
- Memory loss
- Multiple-chemical sensitivities
- New food allergies
- Noise sensitivity
- Numbness and tingling in the limbs
- Rage
- Respiratory infections
- Roving aches and stiffness
- Seizures
- Sore throats
- Stomach pains
- Tremors
- Vertigo

Also, coinfections can cause severe issues as well.

"Ticks can become infected with more than one disease-causing microbe (called coinfection). Coinfection may be a potential problem for humans because ticks that transmit *Borrelia burgdorferi*, the bacterium which causes Lyme disease, often carry and transmit other pathogens, as well." (National Institute of Allergy and Infectious Diseases 2022)

Babesiosis is a common coinfection that can cause:
- Anxiety
- Breathlessness
- Chills
- Decreased appetite
- Depression
- Dizziness
- Fatigue

- Feeling spacey
- Headaches
- High fever
- Muscle pain
- Nausea
- Night sweats

Bartonella, another common coinfection, can cause:
- Anxiety
- Blurred vision
- Fatigue and agitation
- Gut problems
- Headaches
- Heart palpitations
- Joint pain
- Low-grade fever
- Muscle pains
- Nerve irritation
- Panic attacks
- Poor sleep
- Rashes
- Ringing in the ears (tinnitus)
- Sweats

Lyme carditis (heart inflammation) can also be present early as well.

As you can see, the challenges your partner or loved one may face can be enormous.

Learning About Lyme Disease

I would always say I had three priorities. The first was to support what my partner needed to improve her health and the second was to grow my business. Sometimes they flipped.

My third priority was to have an amazing and fun life with her.

That was it.

My adult kids, who I love dearly and who loved her, were on their own. They needed me but didn't rely on me.

My approach was to keep her life as stress-free and fun as possible. If she seemed tired or exhausted, I'd give her space and let her rest. Once I began to study the disease in earnest, I learned that treating and coping with the disease can be all-consuming for chronic Lyme survivors. It can be a daily challenge dealing with the stress, pain, fatigue, and anxiety it causes, and researching ways to ease the pain and the variety of symptoms.

I learned I was mostly ignorant about Lyme disease and how certain things affected it. For example, we once lived in a home that backed up to the woods. I loved seeing the deer come to the deck in the backyard. However, she was more cautious due to the possibility of deer ticks.

Deer ticks.

Wow.

I had no clue.

I knew that deer ticks caused Lyme in many cases, but I had no idea the average deer could have between 2,000 and 4,000 ticks on it!

Since we lived near the woods, the upstairs windowsills were often moldy. One Sunday afternoon, I spent a few hours cleaning up the windowsills across the upstairs. I had no real idea at the time how dangerous mold might be to someone with Lyme, as it inhibits detoxing of the Lyme bacteria.

My partner was very creative and had many great ideas. We liked exploring Washington, DC, where we lived. We walked throughout the entire city on one of our first dates, from Bethesda to the National Zoo. We made many trips like this.

She suggested we document our trips, so we decided to call them our Excellent Adventures. I started riffing on the idea and said we should do one every week. We could create a blog and a podcast detailing everything we did. We decided to start that day.

We had a blast that day, and eventually made it to our favorite restaurant in the District of Columbia.

Blogging, podcasting, and reporting on our trips might have been a little too much to bite off, so that was the only day we had our Excellent Adventure. But it was a lot of fun.

Introduction to Lyme Disease

I had barely heard of Lyme disease when we first met. I don't even recall if I had any reaction when she first told me.

I've had Lyme survivors tell me they have issues with their adrenal glands. I don't think I had given my adrenals any thought. I have since learned that adrenal dysfunction could significantly trigger chronic illness woes. In addition, adrenal insufficiency can weaken the immune system, making it harder for the body to fight Lyme.

I also learned that the Lyme bacteria is very tricky. The actual Lyme bacteria is a spirochete. The corkscrew-shaped bacteria, *Borrelia burgdorferi*, named after the researcher who first isolated the bacterium in 1982, is the same family as the spirochete bacteria that causes syphilis. It is particularly tough to defeat in that it can affect any body organ, including the brain and nervous system, muscles and joints, and the heart.

It can also cross the placenta, and babies can be born with Lyme disease.

As the years went by, I was proud of my partner's determination, courage, and strength. However, my happiness blinded the fact that although life seemed great, she was silently fighting this insidious disease every day. Fighting Lyme disease can be a never-ending battle.

I always said that helping her get her health back was one of my top three goals. However, I soon learned that there was little chance I would cure her. While some people have claimed to be cured of chronic Lyme, the disease wins most of the time until you accept that you have it and build your life around it. We'll discuss this more in the chapter on healing.

Frequently, Lyme disease can go into remission, sometimes for years, and restore normality to your life.

I've met many people who have overcome their Lyme disease by using a mixture of traditional medicine and other Eastern and herbal treatments. Some have been in remission for decades and have lived amazing, healthy, and love-filled lives. Good health, peace, and fun are out there, but you must continue being smart and strong, and do your best to stay as mentally, emotionally, and physically healthy as possible.

In the next chapter, we'll start addressing some of the things you need to know about Lyme disease.

CHAPTER TWO
What You Need to Know about Lyme Disease

Questions to Ponder:
- *What are the things your partner will be concerned about?*
- *What does detox mean, and how does it work?*
- *Why are uneducated health care providers a big problem?*
- *How does the full moon, genetics, and mold play into this?*

When I started learning more about Lyme disease, I was shocked by how little I knew. There were bits of information I retained but in no context.

Here's a partial list of things I learned that chronic Lyme survivors must be conscious of due to how it might affect them:

- Alcohol intake
- Dairy
- Genetics
- Gluten
- Herbal protocols
- Light
- Mold
- Non-native electromagnetic fields (EMF) (e.g., radiofrequency from Wi-Fi and cell phones)
- Sleep
- Sounds
- Soy
- Sugar
- The full moon
- Vitamins

When I was with my partner, my mantra was "pay attention and keep her stress-free." When I first heard of Lyme, I thought that meant fatigue, pain, and maybe anxiety. But she also had amazing energy, was beautiful, brilliant, and very funny.

Everyone loved her kindness, sense of humor, and consideration.

She also had dietary restrictions. When we had pizza, we had to find the best gluten free pizza around. She was also concerned about heavy metals, which meant she did not eat fish that might have mercury. She ate beef and rice when I had sushi.

There were environmental challenges as well. I learned that mold in the basement and around windows might slow healing.

I had no idea that Lyme survivors faced so many daily challenges controlling this insidious disease.

Understanding the Illness

To understand Lyme disease in greater depth, one of the first things I did was go online and purchase every book I could find with the word "Lyme," "chronic illness," or "anxiety" in the title.

Next, I joined a dozen Facebook groups and signed up for mailing lists at LymeDisease.org and other care organizations. I also called everyone I knew whoever uttered the word "Lyme."

After obtaining more information, I was shocked at what I discovered.

I learned it was a constant battle for Lyme survivors to stay on top of treatments, supplements, and relief tools. Many days, all they could do was focus on stopping the pain, addressing the fatigue, and finding relief.

Here are some things you might discover:
- Lyme survivors may feel the balance in the relationship is uneven.
- In a loving relationship, the balance of care shifts. When one partner struggles at work, for example, the other may take a second job. When Lyme disease symptoms arise, the balance will shift.
- She may feel a lot worse than she is telling you.

- Since your partner may sometimes be unable to do some chores, she may think that the workload balance is unfair and feel guilty.
- When one partner is exhausted, the other does the housework and cooks the meals.

It never once occurred to me that these things were an issue. It may not have occurred to you either.

Your partner may have labeled and identified themselves as a "Lyme Sufferer" without hope of being anything else. However, I never saw my partner that way, and you might not see yours that way either.

I saw her wonderful qualities, her beauty, how caring and funny she was. But even though I would share this with her, she might have thought of herself as sick and a burden. Being in pain every day might make it difficult for your partner to believe anything else.

The supplements and herbals? I always saw them as vitamins, not part of a protocol.

So keep all these concerns in mind when your partner is trying to make it through the day, the hour, and sometimes, each minute.

Mold Allergy Can Be Worse Than the Lyme

I didn't realize how devastating mold can be for someone with Lyme. It turns out there are hundreds of thousands of people suffering from mold allergies. People with Lyme are more likely to struggle with mold because their body cannot remove toxins normally. A person with Lyme disease has a damaged immune system, which makes it harder to overcome mold illness. Additionally, the mold illness can stop Lyme treatments from working.

In many cases, the mold allergy is worse than Lyme symptoms up to and including anaphylaxis symptoms in some people.

We moved into a nice house in the suburbs when we brought our families together. Three years after moving in, we discovered mold in the basement.

We brought in a mold remediation specialist, and he confirmed that the mold levels in the basement were very high and needed fixing. Two remediations later, it seemed that the mold was removed. Unfortunately, we had to discard many pieces of furniture and items stored in the basement.

I was personally upset that I had to discard $500 worth of cardboard boxes I saved for the next move. Poor me.

I now know that underlying mold toxicity can prevent Lyme survivors from getting better.

According to Connie Strasheim's book *New Paradigms in Lyme Disease Treatment*:

> Mold toxicity causes patients to develop symptoms from Lyme infections and vice versa, and people with weakened immune systems are far more susceptible to sickness from mold. . . .
>
> Mold illness causes extreme inflammation, called chronic inflammatory response syndrome (CIRS), and when coupled with Lyme disease, symptoms such as fever, headache, and fatigue are exacerbated. Many people are not aware they are simultaneously suffering from CIRS plus Lyme disease. CIRS is a biotoxin illness which is triggered by prolonged exposure to mold.
>
> For most of the population, the body's immune system removes biotoxins through the liver, and people remain healthy with no symptoms. But for those with Lyme, since the immune system is already in a weakened state, the body cannot break the invading biotoxins. Instead, the immune system is supposed to identify a threat and neutralize it through the production of cytokine proteins. . . .
>
> However, with Lyme and other chronic autoimmune disorders, there is an overproduction of cytokine proteins because the body cannot differentiate between the threat and the healthy cells. This produces extreme inflammation. The overproduction of cytokines also causes hormone imbalances. Although the inflammatory response is supposed to protect you from the mold threat, long-term inflammation makes people far sicker than the biotoxins would have made them in the first place. (Strasheim 2016)

Who knew this was such a big part of the Lyme puzzle? I certainly did not.

Coinfections Can Be Worse Than Lyme Disease

Ticks can cause more damage beyond the transmission of Lyme disease. They can also transmit dastardly diseases known as coinfections, although many are just as painful as Lyme disease itself. Many of them are unknown to the doctor you might be seeing. Your doctor may know just enough to recognize that you have Lyme disease, if that.

As an aside, it's hard to test for Lyme disease itself, let alone the coinfections. The infection can hide intracellularly (inside your cells) or inside biofilms designed to evade detection. The inability to properly test for Lyme disease causes some people to retake tests multiple times. Knowing something is wrong but being unable to prove it can cause a lot of anxiety and frustration.

This is a problem.

Unfortunately, these coinfections can coexist in a symbiotic manner with other forms of bacteria, parasites, and viruses that can wreak havoc on your body as well.

The point here is that you need to understand Lyme AND the coinfections. Your partner may have researched coinfections, but if not, be aware of the complications that coinfections can create on top of Lyme disease.

Genetics and Heavy Metals

There are compounding stressors such as heavy metals and coinfections that inhibit the detox. For some, genetic makeup may determine the ability to detox.

Genetics can affect the way the body detoxifies when the Lyme bacteria attacks. Therefore, genetic testing may be needed to create a treatment plan that would work.

Heavy metals such as copper, iron, and zinc can also impact healing. According to the Lyme Warrior website, heavy metals like mold can also inhibit detoxification.

> The most common [non-biologic] heavy metals that can affect the body are Lead, Mercury, Arsenic, Aluminum, and Cadmium. The symptoms for both heavy metal toxicity and chronic toxicity are pretty vague—similar, in fact, to those for Lyme disease. [However,] the most common symptoms are vomiting, nausea, convulsions,

cramping, headaches, breathing problems, impaired motor and cognitive skills, sweating, and more. Some chronic symptoms include depression, fatigue, achy joints, digestive problems, blood sugar issues, menstrual problems, etc.

. . . Heavy metals in the body can begin to interfere with other treatments [because] heavy metals, once built up, will start to form protective layers. This not only prevents and protects the heavy metals themselves, but also other bad guys that may be floating around in your body (i.e., Lyme bacteria). . . .

Treatment for heavy metal toxicity consists primarily of reducing exposure, detoxification, supplements, and therapies such as chelation therapy (with the aid of a doctor). Chelation therapy is the procedure of administering chelating agents into the bloodstream to bind the heavy metals and remove them from the body. Other natural methods can be used as well. (Lyme Warrior 2022)

Chelation is when chemicals, either via IV or oral pills, remove heavy metals and other unhealthy substances from the body.

Most people are not concerned with their heavy metal bodily content. I've never thought about it for a second. I love sushi. I love eating fish and will continue eating fish forever although I know fish might be high in mercury; however, if you have Lyme and are looking for ways to combat the disease, you must get rid of the heavy metals.

Anxiety and Lyme

It's a chicken or the egg issue with anxiety and Lyme. Does chronic Lyme cause anxiety, or does existing anxiety exacerbate the Lyme condition?

Symptoms of anxiety may include:
- A racing heart
- Difficulty concentrating or recalling information
- Difficulty controlling emotions such as worry or fear
- Difficulty sleeping, falling asleep, or sleeping through the night
- Fatigue (or getting fatigued quickly)
- Irritability, dread, panic, or feeling on edge
- Muscle tension, grinding teeth

Finding a Lyme-Literate Medical Doctor (LLMD)

I've come to realize that Lyme healing is a personal, private, and sensitive process that only the person going through it can figure out. Hopefully, you will find a good Lyme-literate medical doctor (LLMD) who can help. I'm amazed at how many doctors still do not understand Lyme.

In most places, Lyme is still mysterious and not well known. This problem becomes even more exacerbated in many states when doctors tell their patients that "Lyme does not exist in our state," when in fact, Lyme has now been found in all 50 states and in many countries around the globe.

Unfortunately, if your partner is ill and you take her to the emergency room, the medical staff may only treat the symptoms and not Lyme disease specifically. It is common for Lyme tests to come back negative even if the patient does have Lyme disease. This is frustrating because you may often find yourself back in the emergency room with your partner. Your partner, who is in chronic pain and suffering from multiple symptoms, will likely be treated to the best of the attending doctor's ability, but the root of the problem, Lyme disease, will still be there.

More health care providers are becoming better informed and mindful of Lyme disease, as well as its coinfections and different treatments. However, the rate of knowledge attainment is dramatically slow. Many survivors would argue that the medical industry overall is horribly slow in learning about the disease, how to diagnose it, and how to care for patients.

It's also important for partners to know that usually whatever your partner is suffering from is not the problem. The problem is Lyme, not the symptom causing the current issue.

Usually.

The Full Moon

Did you know that Lyme survivors may have a difficult time during a full moon? You may have heard your partner mention that her symptoms flare every four weeks, usually when there's a full moon.

It may not be the full moon that's to blame. It could just be the four-week cycle.

The article "Full Moons and Lyme Disease: The Mysterious Correlation" on the website Tired of Lyme references Dr. Joseph Burrascano, an innovator in chronic Lyme treatment. Burrascano observed that many of his chronic Lyme patients' symptoms would "flare" or worsen every four weeks while being treated. He postulated the Lyme bacteria's reproduction cycle was at play here, since antibiotics only kill bacteria during their growth phase.

> Burrascano also observed that the worse a reaction a person with chronic Lyme had during the four-week flare, the higher that person's germ load, and the more ill they were. He goes so far as to suggest that a person still has an active Lyme infection if they feel worse every four weeks and that their treatment should continue.
>
> . . . While it's a credible start by Burrascano, we're not 100 percent certain that the Lyme bacteria's replication cycle is responsible for making people with chronic Lyme feel worse every four weeks. Though it likely is. We also can't conclude that if the Lyme bacteria's replication cycle is to blame for making people with chronic Lyme feel worse every four weeks, those four weeks align with a full moon's four-week cycle, nor that Lyme is triggered to replicate by the full moon. (Tired of Lyme 2021)

It may not be the moon to blame. What is likely happening is that bacteria and parasitic life cycles follow lunar cycles that are driven by how gravitational fields change, as the moon/sun/earth alignment changes every twenty-eight days.

This change in parasite life cycles will affect the human host's immunity. This, in turn, has a likely influence on spirochetes.

How to Be More Helpful

Being healthy is your Lyme survivor's No. 1 priority. It should be a top priority for you, too. It is important to understand that healing from Lyme disease has no timetable. It is essential to know that everyone who suffers from Lyme will recover at their own rate, with their own unique healing protocol. You can't compare your partner's healing journey with anyone else.

You also can't go about it like everything else either. You will need to learn new tools together and not rely on your skills from work, such as scheduling Zoom meetings with her to discuss her health or creating a flow chart. There is no timetable on healing, so don't say, "What are the seven steps we need to do to get to healing in two weeks?" It does not work that way.

Her healing must take its course, and you need to let her lead the way. She knows her body best; you do not.

Remember:

- It is important to know what your partner might be feeling and thinking.
- Your partner didn't ask to get Lyme disease.
- Recovery will take time.
- Recovery is extremely personal. Be patient.
- As she is healing, be sensitive to her needs. Take time to educate yourself about Lyme disease.
- Be there for her. It's different for everyone.
- Listen to her.

I didn't know what healing meant until I learned more about the disease. As a partner, all you can do is get educated, be considerate, and offer support where needed.

You need to do this together in a relationship or it becomes too overwhelming. Life is already overwhelming, even when everything is going your way.

As a partner, you need to make the extra effort to understand your partner's world and what they must do to make it through the day with chronic Lyme.

Questions You Might Want to Ask

- Do you need anything from me?
- Have you done anything recently that is causing you pain?
- What can I do to make your life easier?
- What do I need to know?
- What has helped you move one step up the ladder to wellness?
- What's your symptom list?

- What makes you feel better and what things make you feel worse?
- Which protocols have you tried following? Are you following Buhner or Cowden?
- Which supplements are you taking? Do they help?
- Would you like me to go to the doctor with you?

You're probably not going to help solve all the problems, but at least you'll show that you are aware of what she is going through.

In the next chapter, we'll discuss how stress and other symptoms should be addressed to help your partner heal.

CHAPTER THREE
The Challenges of Understanding Lyme Disease

Questions to Ponder:
- *Is there a treatment for Lyme disease?*
- *Why is it so challenging to be diagnosed?*
- *Why is having Lyme disease so overwhelming?*

When I began understanding how challenging Lyme disease was, I was amazed at how my partner was thriving and not just surviving this horrible disease. But unfortunately, there are better days than others, and you may see your partner in a constant battle to make it through each day.

One day your partner will seem like she is feeling great and almost like her old self—killing it at work, making dinner, cleaning the house, or going for a walk. But then the next day, she may not be able to get out of bed because she overdid it, or her Lyme disease decided to flare up.

The point is to be mindful of how much your partner is doing and pushing it. Also, check in with them and ask if they truly are doing ok and not just saying they are. It not only impacts them, but it also impacts you.

Lyme can be so overwhelming that I want to share some things you might not know, to help you understand the breadth of things your partner might have already spent hundreds of hours researching. Lyme is not readily known throughout the medical profession as much as it should be yet, so your partner has probably had to figure out her own course of treatment, even if, in some cases, she's under the care of a Lyme-literate medical doctor (LLMD).

Everyone who cares about their well-being and health should take control of their health care decisions. If you take control of your own health care experience, you will feel more confident about the choices you make with your health care providers. As a health care advocate, you will be in a better place to ask questions and to share your concerns, preferences, and goals with your health care providers. Also, you will be in a much better position to define what you believe, what you see as living a good quality life, and what matters most to you when it comes to your own health.

It would be beneficial for you to start learning your partner's new vocabulary. For instance, how about comorbidity?

Well, of course, that's the simultaneous presence of two or more diseases or medical conditions in a person. We'll talk more later about the additional coinfections that a tick can transfer. I've never used the word comorbidity in my life, but it could be one that your partner is very familiar with.

If your partner recently discovered that she has Lyme, the information you're about to be exposed to will be overwhelming for several reasons:

- If your partner had Lyme for an extended period, there is no specific cure. Lyme can go into remission, and there are numerous ways to treat it; however, unlike, say, a broken ankle, there is no guaranteed treatment. As you can imagine, this is the source of many frustrations Lyme survivors face. If you break an ankle, you are put in a cast for six weeks. With Lyme, there are many conflicting symptoms, and many don't show up until later. The treatments also vary widely.
- Testing is not perfect. Some tests will detect Lyme; however, the testing may only be 50 percent accurate.
- Antibiotics will help if the disease is detected early enough, and many medical professionals think that's all you need to do. However, antibiotics may be of limited value once the disease has progressed into the chronic stage.

It is common to be misdiagnosed for years before being properly diagnosed with Lyme disease. A reason is that there is no "gold standard" for accurate testing, and physicians who rely only on this testing to make a diagnosis won't get definitive answers. Lyme disease determination is a clinical diagnosis based on signs, symptoms, and history, and by ruling out other diseases as part of a differential diagnosis while using testing as supportive data.

The relief of finally being diagnosed might not last long when you discover how difficult it is to treat Lyme. Unfortunately, there is no universal treatment, or one-size-fits-all protocol.

Many Lyme survivors search far and wide and spend fortunes trying to heal themselves. You can find many alternative treatments within the Lyme community. It may not hurt to try them to see if they will help. Unfortunately, many of these treatments are very expensive, and few of them are covered by health care insurance.

After I wrote a highly downloaded article for Lymedisease.org about being a more supportive partner, many people asked me for medical advice and treatments. I told them I am not qualified to give medical advice, as I am not a doctor. I am a history major with an MBA. I have never had Lyme disease. I just took it upon myself to read many books and articles. My best advice is to contact an LLMD to help.

The next chapter will dive into essential Lyme disease terms that are important to know so you can understand your partner's world better.

CHAPTER FOUR
More Lyme Disease Terms to Know

Questions to Ponder:
- *Do antibiotics cure Lyme disease?*
- *What other ailments can a tick transmit?*
- *Why is detoxing sometimes more challenging than the actual treatment?*

Here is a sample list of terms that your partner is likely already conversant in that you need to be aware of also. Becoming familiar with these terms will help you support your partner and understand her Lyme disease language. As I mentioned before, she may not want you to suggest her treatment approach but to be conversant on how to do so if she wants your advice.

By the way, some outstanding books that go into depth on the topics in this chapter can be found in Appendix A.

Antibiotics, Such as Doxycycline (Doxy)

If a tick bit your partner and you saw the bulls-eye rash, congratulations! You're ahead of the game and probably will be able to tackle Lyme before it becomes too serious. (Note that seeing a bulls-eye rash is not as common as once believed.)

The most common treatment for Lyme is antibiotics such as doxycycline, commonly known as doxy. If your partner gets treatment early enough, the antibiotic is the standard treatment and is often successful. Early detection is vital to limiting complications.

Doxy is prescribed frequently by many doctors, as it also treats anaplasmosis, ehrlichiosis, Rocky Mountain Spotted Fever, and some other coinfections. But dosage recommendations are another reason you should be seeking the treatment of a Lyme-literate medical doctor (LLMD). A regular doctor may give you the two-dose doxy for only a couple of weeks. An LLMD may prescribe more antibiotics and will often combine it with other forms of treatment.

One thing to note is that sometimes people contract Lyme from insects other than ticks, although ticks are the most common transporters. I've heard of people getting bitten by spiders and contracting Lyme as well.

There's a lot of debate about how effective antibiotics are once you have had Lyme for an extended period. Continued use of antibiotics past the initial stage can lead to leaky gut syndrome, persistent yeast infections, and other challenges. However, some people have had some relief using antibiotics in the later stages combined with other treatments. But, again, this is where the LLMD is so critical. An LLMD should be able to help with the side-effects from the antibiotics.

Although it covers many infections, doxy can be rough to handle, and not everyone can. Your LLMD should have other options for you to consider.

Coinfections from Tick Bites

Just when you thought Lyme disease was enough to handle, you may now have coinfections to deal with. Other unique diseases are transmitted via ticks. One of the tricky things is that some of the coinfections are parasitic and some are bacterial. As if the pain, fatigue, anxiety, and stress were not enough, parasites and bacteria might also be living inside the body. With the right treatment, the parasites and bacteria will die, and the body will expel them appropriately.

Some of the most common coinfections are:

- **Anaplasmosis:** An illness that causes fever, muscle aches, and other symptoms. It's an uncommon illness that can affect people of all ages.
- **Babesia:** A parasite, usually transmitted by a tick, that causes an infection of the red blood cells called babesiosis.
- **Bartonella:** A bacteria transmitted from ticks that can cause Lyme-like symptoms. It is known to cause cat scratch disease.
- **Ehrlichia:** A bacteria that causes ehrlichiosis. Symptoms include fever, chills, muscle aches, and an upset stomach.

- **Mycoplasma:** A bacteria that can cause lung, nasal passage, and genital tract infection.
- **Rocky Mountain Spotted Fever:** A bacteria that can be fatal if not treated. Ticks also transmit it. Despite its name, it can be found in the Mid-Atlantic and other areas across the United States.

Treatment of the above complicates matters because it means that more diseases than just Lyme are compromising the immune system. Anything that suppresses the immune system should be removed, like mold, heavy metals, and other toxins.

Detoxing

Killing the Lyme bacteria is not enough. Once the bacteria die, the nasty spirochetes release endotoxins into the blood. Detoxification is crucial to cleansing the blood by removing impurities.

Before discussing detoxification, I want to present another common term—binding, or binding agent. When the bacteria die off, binding agents clean up the bacteria and their endotoxic byproducts like ammonia, so they won't get reabsorbed by the gut lining.

Here are some common binders your partner may be using:

- **Activated Charcoal:** Activated charcoal is great because it works well and is very inexpensive. It might also be a subtler method of detox than other methods.
- **Alka Seltzer Gold:** Reduces the pain related to the detox and the herxing (more about the Herxheimer effect later in the book) that occurs when the bacteria die off.
- **Apple Cider Vinegar:** When mixed with hot water, lemon, and raw honey, it's an excellent way to start the cleanse in the morning.
- **Bentonite Clay:** A common ingredient in cat litter, it has been used for centuries around the globe to help with detox.
- **Chlorella:** A blue-green algae commonly used to remove heavy metals from the body, such as mercury.
- **Coffee Enema:** It is what it sounds like. The caffeine from the coffee goes to the liver, creates more bile and glutathione, and aids in the elimination.

- **Epsom Salt Bath:** Sulfates and magnesium in the Epsom salt increase the liver's ability to produce bile, like some other detox agents. The bath can also help reduce stress and anxiety, often the result of Lyme disease.
- **Infrared Saunas:** Much more powerful than a traditional sauna, the infrared sauna can penetrate deeper into tissues to eliminate toxins. Like the Epsom salt bath, it can also reduce stress and anxiety.
- **Ionic Foot Bath:** Currents processed in the bath remove toxins from the feet. The currents are modified to disrupt pathogens, parasites, and candida cells.
- **Lemon Water:** Perhaps the least expensive way to detox, lemons stimulate bile production to help cleanse the liver.
- **Oil Pulling:** Lyme bacteria can reside in oral and gum tissues, so patients need to be careful even when getting simple dental work! Several products on the market can gently help with this.
- **Tea:** The Lyme bacteria works very hard to defend itself against antibiotics. Certain teas can break down the biofilms that the bacteria produce to protect themselves.
- **Vitamin C:** Can help if your immune system is compromised.

Herbal Protocols

A common approach to treating late-stage or chronic Lyme is with herbals. If your partner has boxes or cabinets filled with plastic bottles of natural remedies, she probably is following an herbal protocol. There are several herbal protocols available. One of the most popular was created by master herbalist Stephen Buhner. His book can be found in Appendix A.

Here are some common herbals:
- Cat's Claw
- Cnidium Root
- Corydalis
- Herb Pharm Eleuthero
- Japanese Knotweed
- Milk Thistle
- Olive Leaf

- Safflower
- Scutellaria
- Sophora Root
- Wormwood Flower

Each herbal addresses something specific, and your partner has probably researched what that is.

Herxheimer Reaction (Herxing)

Herxing is a typical but painful response to the bacteria being killed off in your body when you're detoxing. When too much herxing takes place, it could mean that the amount of toxins released is more than the body can handle.

It can be very unpleasant and can last hours and sometimes days. If it's too strong, it can also signify that the treatment to kill off the Lyme bacteria might be too aggressive. Herxing can also cause stress on the internal organs.

In the next chapter, we'll discuss some of the neurological issues related to Lyme that you should be aware of.

CHAPTER FIVE
Neurological Concerns

Questions to Ponder:
- *Why is chronic Lyme called "The Great Imitator"?*
- *How does Lyme impact normal brain functions?*
- *How do you help keep stress to a minimum?*

[NOTE: The purpose of this book is not to suggest medical treatment or care. It's to help partners, family members, and friends be aware of how Lyme disease may affect their loved one. Thus, we won't be going into a lot of detail in this chapter about how Lyme may affect brain activities. If you need more information, please see a Lyme-literate medical doctor (LLMD) or neurologist. You can also refer to some of the books listed in Appendix A.]

Lyme is known as the "Great Imitator" because its symptoms might resemble other diseases. The Lyme bacteria can impact almost every organ in the body and replicate other diseases.

It can attack the central nervous system and affect brain functions in some cases. In more severe cases, you'll need to make special accommodations.

According to Dr. Olga Syritsyna, 15 percent of Lyme cases affect the central nervous system when it becomes neurological Lyme. (Syritsyna 2022)

Some symptoms might be:
- Dizziness
- Brain fog
- Confusion
- Decreased ability to concentrate
- Depersonalization
- Difficulty remembering words
- Dissociation

- Feet numbness and lack of strength
- Impaired abstract reasoning
- Lack of verbal fluency
- Loss of memory
- Panic attacks
- Poor balance
- Short-term memory loss
- Tinnitus
- Vibration inside the head
- Visual snow
- Weakness in the legs

According to Dr. Todd Maderis, the bacteria that causes Lyme disease and its associated infections can affect the central, peripheral, and autonomic nervous systems.

One result is postural orthostatic tachycardia syndrome (POTS). Maderis explains how POTS occurs: "The heart rate will increase when someone changes position, from lying or sitting to standing. POTS is very common in late-stage Lyme disease since the autonomic nervous system does not maintain tone in blood vessels causing a drop in blood pressure." (Maderis 2022)

It is essential to have a personal neurological Lyme disease treatment plan, as the manifestation of the disease varies so much across patients. The symptoms have different stages, and various body systems are affected.

One other quick note: When Lyme affects the central nervous system, the symptoms might show up like multiple sclerosis (MS). You may need to check with a specialist if concerned.

Why Stress Needs to Be Reduced

Environmental concerns, trauma, and stress can make it more difficult for the body to destroy the Lyme bacteria. When the body is fighting the causes of the stress, attacking the Lyme bacteria can be a challenge.

According to the article "Full Moons and Lyme Disease" on TiredofLyme.com:

> When the body is exposed to a high-stress situation, it has an innate response to allow it to cope—the flight or fight response. The flight or fight response activated in those with Lyme Disease appears to cause more stress on the body than the initial reason that caused the high stress in the first place. You have the adrenal glands being called upon, and in those with Lyme, adrenal fatigue is likely already present.
>
> Glucose levels rise, or at least they're called upon to do so, and a person with Lyme may be dealing with Lyme-induced glucose problems. The glucose needed to fuel muscles during a fight or flight response may not be there for consumption, or may be distorted, which may be the cause for shaky or weak muscles. The body also releases a lot of hormones during a high-stress situation which may also not be available for use because Lyme can affect the endocrine system.
>
> All of these imbalances will not allow the flight or fight response to work in the way evolution has intended it to, and as an alternative result, leave a person with Lyme feeling all out of whack for potentially a day or more. High-stress situations are very taxing on a body without Lyme Disease, and a body with Lyme Disease really takes the hit. (Tired of Lyme 2021)

In the next chapter, we'll meet some people with Lyme disease who live powerful, mission-driven lives.

CHAPTER SIX
Stories of Lyme Survivors and How You Can Make a Difference

Questions to Ponder:
- *What are some things you can do to make a difference in the Lyme community?*
- *How can you promote more awareness of Lyme disease?*
- *What are some of the challenges people with chronic Lyme face?*

I had no idea that such a large community struggled with Lyme disease. The Lyme survivors I met in the Lyme communities were incredibly helpful in understanding their daily challenges. After listening to and getting to know some Lyme survivors, I wanted to make a difference. Staring at the pile of books I had already read on my nightstand, I decided to give them away to other people with Lyme who might get some value from them.

This decision changed the course of my life.

There's a Hebrew expression *Tikkun olam*, which means "Repair the World." A big part of the Jewish faith revolves around making the world you live in better. There is more suffering in the Lyme world than I had ever known.

I originally purchased the books to learn what I needed to help my partner recover. I soon learned many people could benefit from the books. I started gifting the books in the Lyme Facebook groups.

The response to my gifting was overwhelming. I learned that many people with Lyme disease live challenging lives. Not only do they have to live with the effects of the disease, but many also deal with family members and friends who don't believe they are ill. Also, treatment is often not covered by insurance.

I was able to spread some kindness by the simple act of giving away a book that might help someone. If I only had one copy and received numerous requests for the book, I went online and ordered a copy for everyone who asked. Spending a couple of bucks to help someone learn about treatments or strategies to recover was well worth it. If I could impact one life, it was worth it.

As a successful podcaster, I like to say, "If one person is listening to my podcast, one person is listening to my podcast." The same thing applied here. If I could brighten one person's day, I was brightening one person's day.

Making a Difference

I met many courageous people who overcame their initial struggles and rediscovered their life's mission. Some of these people wrote books, and some created nonprofit entities to help others attain a higher quality of life while recovering from Lyme disease.

I have been able to converge two of the most essential things in my life—my business, and my understanding of Lyme disease—on my *Sales Game Changers Podcast*. On my podcast, we discuss topics designed to help sales professionals take their careers to the next level. We frequently discuss the idea of understanding your "why" or your life's mission. The concept of "why" was made famous in a TED talk by Simon Sinek.

In the Lyme community, I met three people who saw an opportunity to create a new, positive life for themselves after conquering their Lyme disease. They have gone on to help and promote Lyme awareness. I brought them all together on a special podcast episode in June 2021. The complete transcript can be found at: www.salesgamechangerspodcast.com/mission.

The panel featured Gregg Kirk, author of *The Gratitude Curve* and founder of the nonprofit Lyme patient fund the Ticked Off Foundation. I had read *The Gratitude Curve*, and that's how I got to meet him.

Tanya Hoebel is vice president of The Lyme Center in Chico, California, and cofounder of the popular Lyme Conquerors Mentoring Lyme Warriors Facebook group. She's also co-host of the *Integrated Lyme Solutions* podcast.

And J. P. Davitt is the founder of Lymefriends and the author of *Lymebook: A Journey to Becoming One Day Better*.

I share each of their stories from the *Sales Game Changers Podcast* in the following sections.

Gregg's Story

It started when I was at my worst. I was at the point where I wanted to die, and I just wasn't dying. One night I had more or less a heart attack as a result of that picc line jab, and at that point, I thought, okay. I started to pray to have God take me. I'd led a great life up to that point, I thought. I wasn't going to do it by my own hand, so it didn't happen. It was one of these weird situations where I wanted to die, but I kept hanging around.

Then I started looking inward. Why am I still here, and why have I gone through this? Is this some kind of weird karma thing? Did I deserve this? Did I kill someone in a past life? Why am I going through all this mental and physical punishment? Then after I had that night, I let everything go, and I started looking at my life in a different way.

I more or less got jettisoned from the corporate world and went through a period of time where I was making quite a bit of money, to I wasn't. I decided I'm just going to start doing nonprofit work and fly on the trapeze without a net. It was some wild times. I wasn't making a lot of money. To be able to make some money, I was actually trained by Dr. (William Lee) Cowden. He developed a protocol, and it's one of the protocols that helped me get better. I was lucky enough to be invited to be trained with fifteen doctors. It just made no sense. It was just one of these weird coincidences.

I learned energy healing before that, so I opened my clinic in Connecticut in 2017, and I started doing that for a living along with the foundation work. The more I started focusing on that type of work, the more I realized this is why I'm here.

During the dark days, I thought, why am I going through this? Then a couple of friends talked to me about that, and they said, "You know that healers are usually the wounded ones, and they're the ones that need to experience it so that they can better help people heal." That was when I realized my why right there.

Lyme disease is in every state, whether people get infected in those states. In a state like Hawaii, it's 70 percent military personnel. They're getting infected in different parts of the world and coming to Hawaii where they say there's no Lyme disease, but all these people are sick. We raised awareness, but instantly within the first year, I realized a bigger problem that my nose is being shoved into: There is a patient care problem. People have no money, and they're not getting diagnosed properly. When they finally are, they're not getting the proper care. Even going to an LLMD is a better situation, but a lot of times they're not the best people either.

I took a step back and I thought, if I had a billion dollars, what would I do? I thought I would create a health care system, like an insurance system that funded treatment because most of the treatments that worked for me were not covered by insurance—the herbal treatments and so forth. I thought, I don't need to wait until I'm a billionaire, I can start a foundation, a nonprofit that [lets] people come to us. They get qualified through some documentation, and we give them monthly stipends.

It started by us running after some other groups that give thousands of dollars to patients. But we quickly found out that once the word got out that The Ticked Off Foundation Inc. was giving away free money, we became overwhelmed. [Now] we give out what I call microgrants. We get people who are qualified to sit down with every single patient for at least an hour-long chat. They find out their level of need and agree on what's the best thing for them. Then we give them a microgrant every month.

After that, I wrote *The Gratitude Curve*. In the middle of all this, I realized that my mission was to help people avoid what I went through or at least guide them through it. (Kirk, Sales Game Changers Podcast, 2021)

Tanya's Story

I'm a good person. I feel like I do the right thing. But it just felt like time and time again, things were not looking my way. Then again, here I am, set with this horrible debilitating illness, and I had no explanation. When I was nearing the end of my treatment, which was about nine years into my illness, I could for the first time see the light at the end of the tunnel. I really had some faith that I was going to get better.

By now, my brain had been functioning at a more optimal level than it had been for the last nine years. I really had some time to sit back and reflect on the last decade of my life. Because of the lack of knowledge of my disease that caused me to get sick, I was the lucky one who got the bullseye rash but I didn't know what it meant. I think that there needs to be so much more awareness about it.

I always jokingly say that I can be a therapist, a pharmacist, and a doctor; unfortunately, I don't have the credentials for that. Because you truly need to be your own advocate when you're dealing with Lyme because Western medicine failed me time and time again. Knowing the hundreds of thousands of dollars that I'd spent during this Lyme journey, how it had truly financially ruined me, I didn't let it physically or emotionally ruin me because I continued to fight back.

I thought, how can I possibly allow another human being to go through even one day of what I've gone through over the last nine years? I knew somehow that I had to help. I didn't know how or what, but I thought all of this knowledge I've learned over all these years has to be good for something. That's when I decided that my new mission in life needed to be to educate and advocate for those that are too sick to do it themselves. That's why I do what I do.

I've always considered myself a very chatty girl, a very bubbly girl, very outgoing, and never really had a negative thing to say about anything in life because everything happens for a reason. But in my darkest days during my journey, I actually contemplated suicide. I thought there was no other way to end my pain. I'm so thankful that I found another resource to end my suffering. It truly does tend to make you feel a little more grateful for all the little things in life, even though I never felt ungrateful. I think maybe I took the birds chirping outside for granted, whereas I used to not be able to go outside to hear them.

Things like that really did change my way of thinking. It proved to me also that someone on top of the world emotionally, financially and at the top of their career like I was prior to Lyme can in one moment lose it all. I could have been one of those people homeless on the streets that you see roaming around, and you often wonder why they're there. That is what Lyme disease does physically, emotionally, and financially.

Because this positive person contemplated suicide at one point, I thought I've got to do something. I've got to make a difference. That is when I became so involved in advocating for Lyme. I run a nonprofit organization called The Lyme Center. It's based out of Chico, California, and our mission is to educate and advocate for Lyme. We do fundraisers to help raise money. This past spring, we were able to have a great significant number of patients tested through one of the well-known labs and we were able to pay for that by the donations and the fundraisers that we get.

I'm also the cofounder of an incredible mentoring group. This group has proved to be more than I ever dreamt it to be in such a short amount of time. We offer lots of treatment options and just help educate them on so many different levels of Lyme because there are so many facets of it. We do bimonthly Zoom calls. Last night we had our first healing concert through vibrations and sound. We're coming up with new and incredible ways every week to help all of those struggling through Lyme.

I even managed to find time to co-host a weekly podcast, *Integrative Lyme Solutions*. I do it with an integrative doctor, very generous with his time, Dr. Michael Karlfeldt. Right now, our podcast is leading interviews of those that haven't beaten Lyme. We talk about where their journey started, when they got sick, how sick, how they were treated, and where they are now. It's been another great way to add those relationships into my community. I love it. (Hoebel, Sales Game Changers Podcast, 2021)

J. P.'s Story

When I was sick, I dreamt of a platform that would allow sick people to connect more easily with one another. Facebook had evolved at this point, and it is a helpful tool, but I imagined a social platform that was more like online dating for wellness. This tool I created evolved into the idea of "crowdcuring" Lyme disease and chronic illness, and eventually evolving again into the Lymefriends Healing app and the Lymefriends platform. I fund my ideas through my financial advisory practice, which also helped me to create a sales niche to converge my two passions.

I did realize that, for the first time, I was really speaking without a filter. I projected this idea out to the universe, and apparently the universe was holding me accountable. Ever since, I've been a man on a mission. I spoke it into existence. I meditated on it. Apparently, the universe approved, and I kept speaking ideas and thoughts to the world no matter how crazy they seemed to be. All the ducks keep lining up, whether it's funding or the tools I need.

I was with the banks for fifteen years, and I opened up my own practice. I'm the president of Good Life Financial of Pittsburgh. I have a big Venn diagram on the front of my building that says "Health plus wealth equals freedom." I created an interactive health and wealth advisory practice, and my passion became my niche.

Regarding health care, Lyme disease is a passion. I have Lymefriends and I work tightly and closely with Tanya as a partner on the Lyme Conquerors Mentoring Lyme Warriors Facebook page. We host mentoring calls on Lymefriends. It is a platform that acts like a dashboard for people with Lyme disease to go to, a one-stop shop for all resources. I collect resources without worrying about any competition and bring everything together to help them finance sooner.

Whenever I was sick and had to streamline my efficiency with my body, it really taught me a lot about processes. Learning a lot about this process as I carried that over to health care, I was able to form a goal to help with Lyme disease.

My goal really, in the grand picture, is to change the literacy and vocabulary of health care using technology. Right now, I'm testing, retesting, improving technology all the time, trying to help people become one day better. It's undoubtedly high-risk and high reward, but it has certainly given me a very clear purpose. (Davitt, Sales Game Changers Podcast, 2021)

I was so inspired by the messages that Gregg, Tanya, and J. P. discussed that I decided to do more podcasts bringing Lyme success stories that converged with the sales lessons we were sharing. I was introduced to a sales leader and solar energy business owner named T. J. Nelson, based in Las Vegas. T. J. was afflicted with Lyme disease and has continued to perform at a high level. His story can be heard at www.salesgamechangerspodcast.com/tjnelson.

T. J.'s Story

Lyme essentially weakens the immune system; it gets in throughout your whole body and then that causes a host of other issues where other things can take hold more easily. Then the Lyme causes a lot of damage. Right now, what's interesting is that my test results show that the Lyme isn't really that big of a deal anymore, but there's been so much damage, and now I have autoimmune issues and all this other stuff that came with it. Chronic Lyme is when Lyme causes long-term problems for the person.

Before I had Lyme, I was a machine. I had energy all day long. I was already eating healthy and all that, and I was just pure obsessed. I'm a more type-A kind of guy, hyper-competitive. If someone was ahead of me in sales, I literally couldn't sleep right until I was ahead of them. I was just going super hard. I had a lot of charisma, and I could go all day long, every day, on machine mode.

After the Lyme, I couldn't even work for a year and a half. I couldn't do anything, and everything fell apart. I couldn't work a real job or business. I didn't really know if I was going to make it for eight months or if I was going to die. It was so rough. I had to use my willpower to get up, and I had to sell to people purely based on mechanics and strategy. Because I felt so bad, I had zero charisma. And it was weird because I'd have the strategy and I would sign people up using the tactics and the techniques, but they would never talk to me again, like they didn't like me. I went from selling with charisma and energy to having no energy or charisma. So I had to learn how to sell purely based on mechanics and strategy.

I would go to an appointment, come back home, lay in bed, get up, go to another appointment, come home, and lay back in bed.

It was a nightmare.

Basically, before, I was able to sell with energy and charisma and all that stuff, and then afterward, it was just pure survival sales mechanics. So that's how I'd have to sell deals.

I was in a lot of denial, too, because in door-to-door sales it's all mindset. I was overpowered. I was still in that mode to just push through it all, which hurt me more. It was really hard for me to learn how to surrender to that and flow with it versus trying to overcome it like I was used to being able to do before getting an illness.

One of the best analogies is, let's say you have a Lamborghini, and maybe before you get sick, you can drive at 120 miles an hour, then you get sick, and you can only go 35. It can be frustrating, and you might try and drive faster than that, and then you're going to hurt yourself. But you can still get to the destination. You just might have to do it a little differently. You might not be able to take the freeway. It can be frustrating not to drive 120 miles an hour, but you still have to just drive.

Some days are worse than others.

I go to bed at 11:15 p.m. every night. I meditate every single day. I don't sleep with my phones in my room. I don't watch TV. There's a TV back there. I don't know why I bought it because I never turn it on. Then every morning, I wake up. I don't check my phone right away. I do my health routine. I drink my smoothie. I go for a walk in the sun, and then I check my phone. I have a cook, and she cooks all of my meals, so I don't eat anything but those meals. I have to live a very strict life. It's meditation, bed at 11:15, morning routine every day, eating only healthy food every single day, taking the supplements, and everything to keep that state alive.

It is hard for me to hear people complaining, especially in the solar industry. When I used to sell five years ago, it was way harder, and the pay was way less. So when someone's complaining, there are so many people in this world that would do anything to be in your position. But in a salesperson's mind, it's easy to get trapped into that because there are so many things that go wrong.

It's almost like one of your jobs as a sales professional is to learn how to generate positive emotions and beliefs. That's part of your job. There's always going to be something happening that's chaotic, wrong, your customer cancels, there's always that. You have to become that person that it just rolls off you, especially if you're knocking on doors. (Nelson, Sales Game Changers Podcast, 2021)

T. J. is a high-performing professional, which leads to the question of being able to work. It is possible to work and treat Lyme symptoms, but not everyone can. The fatigue, stress, and pain could make it very difficult to work a standard corporate job or a retail position where you need the energy to interact with customers all day.

Some LLMDs encourage their Lyme survivors to work as much as possible to keep their minds and bodies fresh. It could also keep their minds off their disease, which can be helpful.

In the next chapter, we'll discuss some of the little things you can do to make your partner's life easier.

CHAPTER SEVEN
The Little Things You Can Do to Make Everyone's Life Easier

Questions to Ponder:
- *How can you help with housework, school activities, and chores?*
- *How are intimacy, work, parenting, and alone time impacted?*
- *How can you improve your communication and relationship?*
- *Why do some people not believe chronic Lyme is a real thing?*

Being in a relationship takes a lot of energy and time and care.

Being in a relationship with your partner or family member with Lyme disease can be complicated.

Unfortunately, many relationships fall apart when one person has chronic illness and pain. Both of you may feel walking away would be easier at times. However, continuing to foster healthy communication is crucial for support, guidance, and love.

Here are some things you can do:
- Give your partner frequent compliments.
- Remind them of what they can still do and don't focus on what they can't.
- Remind them that you are still attracted to them and will always love them.
- Remind them that they are important and try to encourage them.
- Talk about your memories but learn how to move on with Lyme disease together.
- Tell your partner why they are important not just to you but to others in the family.

There's an expression that if you have your health, you can do and think of anything. When you don't, you can only focus on one thing.

When I joined some Facebook Lyme disease groups, I was stunned by how many women and men felt guilty about burdening their families. I would always reply with a comment that many partners don't identify them with their disease, like a woman calling herself "Lyme Lucy," for example. I never saw my partner that way. I always saw her as beautiful, funny, brilliant, and kind.

Your partner may think that you resent them for having the disease. Make sure they know that isn't true.

Sometimes I found myself catching glimpses of my partner and reminding myself of how lucky I was to have her in my life.

Do the same.

I recall a family event we attended. A family member looked at her for the first time and said, "Oh my, you're so pretty. We need someone like you in the family!"

I tried to make sure my partner knew she was important. When she would drive, I would glance over at her and scan her from head to toe. She was not only beautiful on the outside but even more beautiful on the inside. When we would sit on the couch and watch television, I would gently touch her to stay connected.

I've learned that many Lyme survivors feel guilty for taking so much time, energy, and perhaps money to take care of themselves and find a successful treatment. Often, they feel guilty also for neglecting their children, friends, and other family members.

Please be conscious of that.

Your partner may also have guilt and sadness for primarily thinking about recovery and nothing else.

Also, know that she may think she's not the person she once was. In many situations, the effects of Lyme become apparent when the rigors of being a parent, a partner, and an employee converge. Women's responsibilities as mothers, coupled with the devastating challenges of fighting the disease, are overwhelming.

Believe in Them, Even Though Others May Not

I've learned that many Lyme survivors often do not get the support they need from family members and friends. This is due to the lack of the disease's recognition. Even the Centers for Disease Control (CDC) and the Infectious Diseases Society of America (IDSA) don't acknowledge that chronic Lyme is a valid disease. So why would family and friends? If a family member is unsure about what their loved one is suffering from, and they search "Is chronic Lyme disease real?" one of the first things they'll see is this Wikipedia entry:

> Chronic Lyme disease is the name used by some people with "a broad array of illnesses or symptom complexes for which there is no reproducible or convincing scientific evidence of any relationship to *Borrelia burgdorferi* infection" to describe their condition and their beliefs about its cause. Both the label and the belief that these people's symptoms are caused by this particular infection are generally rejected by medical professionals, and the promotion of chronic Lyme disease is an example of health fraud.
>
> Chronic Lyme disease in this context should not be confused with genuine Lyme disease, a known medical disorder caused by infection with *Borrelia burgdorferi*, or with post-treatment Lyme disease syndrome, a set of lingering symptoms that may persist after successful treatment of infection with Lyme bacteria. (Wikipedia 2022).

The above is why so many people are being misdiagnosed, undiagnosed, and neglected. It causes a great deal of harm to those suffering from Lyme disease and other tick-borne illnesses.

The last thing any Lyme survivor needs to deal with is family members who question anything about their illness. Since it's so expensive to treat chronic Lyme, many survivors depend on family members, perhaps parents, to help with expenses. Sometimes these survivors will hear from other family members that the illness is psychosomatic, and they are putting an unfair burden on the parent who is paying the bills. This can lead to discord.

Resentment against Lyme Disease

Another challenge is acknowledging and accepting that the Lyme survivor may not be the person they once were. They may never be again.

They may think you resent them for having this disease.

Their attention and energy may only be focused on finding a treatment that will help them heal.

The lack of attention and the reality of knowing this person you love is not the same can put a huge strain on any relationship.

I've learned that many relationships have unfortunately ended because of this. It is important to remind your Lyme survivor that they are a priority to you. Spending time sharing how much you care and love them for who they are now will make a huge difference in your relationship.

Actively communicating and strengthening your relationship can be challenging, but worth it.

Don't let the disease win.

In the next chapter, we'll discuss how to ensure your family continues to thrive.

CHAPTER EIGHT
Covering Family Activities

Questions to Ponder:
- *What do you do when your partner is too fatigued to make it to school functions?*
- *What do you tell the kids and other family members?*
- *How does your partner feel about missing school or family functions?*

I've learned that many Lyme survivors struggle with managing their children and their afterschool activities. Usually, the mother is the default manager of the children's activities and coordinates the scheduling, carpooling, and other details. However, when fatigue sets in and energy levels are low, she may not balance all that needs to get done. This may include attending school functions, helping with homework, or even putting the kids to bed.

If the partner cannot take off from work, it might be necessary to explain to the kids that certain things, such as both parents attending after-school activities, may not happen. This is where other family members or friends may need to proactively step in and support the kids' activities.

Unfortunately, in some situations, family members and friends may unknowingly blame the Lyme survivor for not attending these activities. You might need to stand up to defend your partner, and to explain what Lyme is and how it's affecting her.

Maybe buy them a copy of this book?

Again, not many people understand the disease and the impact it can cause. Whenever I ask someone if they are familiar with Lyme disease and they say they are, I always ask if they are intimately familiar or somewhat familiar. It allows me to explain it in more detail to them.

Remember also that your partner is not happy about this. Frequently, the disease rears its ugly head when your partner is most active with work, kid activities, or other stressful situations.

Your partner will not be happy if she misses school plays, sporting events, and parent-teacher conferences. You're going to have to make it a priority to be there. And you can't treat it like an obligation. Take joy in it. Make sure your schedule works so that you're able to be at everything.

Plus, it will mean a lot to your kids. I made it a point to be at every kid's activity. When I would drive my youngest daughter to school, I would sometimes stay in the lobby to make phone calls. I remember one of the teachers came up to me once and said, "Just wanted to let you know that we all notice how much you're here."

I've learned that many Lyme survivors feel guilty that they cannot attend all their kids' things. And if your kids are also infected, which is not uncommon, the burden increases. Let her know that you're on top of these things, so it's less of a burden.

Being a Super Dad

If you have children, be conscious that your partner may not feel like participating in school functions, sporting events, or family events due to fatigue. This can take an emotional toll on everyone in the family. In many cases, even in "egalitarian" households, the mother handles much of the children's activities, such as extracurricular activities, sports, and playdates. If the fatigue and pain are too high, those activities might get shunted.

There may be times when you must go above and beyond in your role to help the household and life flow efficiently. This will help decrease your partner's stress, the family's stress, and yours over time.

Other ideas could be to take the kids to appointments, play with them at home, help with homework/projects and meals, spend time asking how their day was, or drop them off at friends' houses. Perhaps arrange your work schedule to help with carpooling.

- Discuss your kid's activities with your partner and ask her what she'd like you to do.

- Get to know your kid's teachers. Email them on occasion to let them know you're paying attention.
- Make it a point to attend parent-teacher meetings. Get on your school's email list and put these meetings on your calendar.
- Put your kids' activities on your calendar so that you can be there, not just to help your partner but to show your kids you care.
- Show up at your kids' sporting events.
- Volunteer to coach their sports teams.

Make these things a priority. Working together as a family unit will make changes flow smoother if your partner cannot participate due to a Lyme flare.

In the next chapter, we'll discuss ways to step up your game.

CHAPTER NINE
Step Up Your Game Because She Deserves It

Questions to Ponder:
- *How can you recognize when you're overwhelmed?*
- *How can you deal with not being able to do enough?*
- *How do you continue to support your partner when you don't think you're making a difference?*

It may feel that you are not doing enough to help. Check in with your partner to see if there is anything else you can do. If so, you may have to step up your game a bit.

You committed to supporting each other in sickness and in health. Now more than ever is the time to honor this.

In total, my partner and I had five kids between us. My youngest daughter left for college in 2020, and then we were empty nesters.

Once all the kids left, my priorities became growing my business, supporting my partner to become healthier, and planning our future. When the COVID lockdown occurred, my focus shifted to making my business work from a virtual perspective, like many people I knew.

My company primarily conducted live events for sales professionals in the Washington, DC, region. Suddenly, live events were not happening. I shifted our programs and events to virtual. Luckily, I had a subscription to GoToWebinar. I dusted it off and started conducting daily webinars for sales teams.

I had no problem getting sales authors and speakers on upcoming shows. Many of them spoke for a living. Now, they were looking for places to speak, and virtual was the only real option. So we started doing webinars every day of the week. I would conduct them from my home office.

As the pandemic wore on, I would go downstairs to my office by 7:00 a.m. and sometimes work until 10:00 p.m. I wanted to grow my business as quickly as I could. I learned that treating Lyme disease was expensive. Many doctors who treat Lyme do not take insurance. Although they may generally charge acceptable hourly rates, patient costs often rise because the doctor must see the patient for longer visits, and there is a high amount of overhead due to disability claims. I wanted to make sure I was generating enough income from my business to afford the best treatments available. It was not until later that I realized how difficult it was to find a good Lyme doctor, and it was stressful.

My partner was loved by everyone I knew. All my family members, friends, and colleagues enjoyed spending time with us and looked forward to hanging out with her.

In the early days of the formation of my company, the Institute for Excellence in Sales, she was a huge help. On one particularly troublesome day, she was a savior.

Each month, we held events for sales leaders and teams at companies such as Salesforce, Oracle, and IBM. When we first started, we held them at a beautiful conference center in a major business area near Washington, DC, known as Tysons Corner. The building housed USA Today as its major tenant.

One day in July 2014, we had our biggest registration to date—over 150 people. We also had a couple of interesting things happen. For the first time ever, we ordered scrambled eggs for the main breakfast food offering. Since this facility did not have a cooking staff in the kitchen, there was nothing left to serve once the eggs ran out. The first ten people in line must have thought they were at an all-you-could-eat buffet and finished off all the eggs. There were none left! I turned ashen pale when I realized we would run out of food.

Secondly, the audio-video system was not working. Our speaker, a telemarketing expert, was set up and ready to go. But even though this was a world-class conference center, we could not get the AV to work!

And finally, since our event director was on vacation, we had a backup person create name tags, which were a big deal for us. Most people started arriving around 7:00 a.m. for breakfast. The backup person was late, and the name tags did not arrive until 7:30 a.m.

Ok, so we were out of eggs, the AV was not working, and we did not have name tags. My brain was going crazy. I expected to have to shut down the company that afternoon. I remember hiding in a corner, trying to collect myself.

My partner managed the registration table like a pro. She kindly welcomed people and told them that she would get them their name tags as soon as they arrived. Then she came over and consoled me. She knew how crestfallen I was at that moment.

Miraculously, the AV started working, and the name tags appeared! We were still without food, but the catering manager found some pastry. The day turned out to be a huge success. It was very stressful but worked out well in the end.

Managing Stress and Healing

Until I started doing research and reading about the disease, I thought that reducing my partner's stress was all I needed to do and that it would be enough.

I was ignorant, and you may be as well.

I thought by taking a methodological approach to healing her, it would eventually happen.

I was wrong.

Some of the **best doctors on the planet** have limited ideas about how to treat Lyme, which is why so many survivors have become detectives, relying on others on chat boards and Facebook groups to share information about what worked and what did not. They create detailed journals tracking every supplement they take and how their body responded. They try new things in different doses at different times of the day to understand what may or may not work.

Healing from Lyme is a personal matter. You have no idea how your partner's body is feeling at any time. She may seem energized and pain-free, but she may be hiding how she's really feeling, perhaps willing mind over matter.

Many men, like me, like to solve our partner's problems prescriptively: identify the problem, create a plan of attack, and then execute the solution. We try to make it as simplistic as possible. That was my approach to curing her Lyme disease. Let's get a doctor, perhaps a functional or integrative medicine specialist, and let's see how it goes. Follow a plan, and, hmm, let's see, be cured in a few weeks. Then we can do a long weekend by the lake.

Lyme does not work that way.

There are no easy solutions.

You will be naïve in thinking that you can cure your partner's Lyme. She is thinking about it all the time and is working hard to control it. How could you, with limited knowledge, even begin to believe that you could?

The main thing that stressed me was not being able to solve her medical problems. You also may be in the same boat I was.

Take Care of You First

To properly support your partner, you need to take care of yourself. As they say on airplanes, put your own oxygen mask on first.

As I started getting deeper into my understanding of chronic Lyme, I realized I had some things I needed to take care of. You may have similar things to address.

Your partner may think she is causing you stress. She's not. What causes you stress is your own doing. Maybe you're not making as much money as you'd like, and you're living too tightly. Maybe your business is struggling because you're not focusing on the right things. Maybe there are some personal relationships that need closure.

I took some time to discover what was really blocking me from unparalleled success. And what I discovered was life changing.

Now, understand. I was doing well. I'd had close to a million interactions with my *Sales Game Changers Podcast* over the years. I had world-class companies such as Amazon Web Services, Red Hat Software, Net App, Salesforce, and others participating in our programs. The top sales authors and speakers would always accept my invitations to come to

Washington to speak. My company was on an upswing, but I was not always comfortable with our success.

I used this opportunity to understand the cause of any stress I might have. I went back and read journals I filled over the past five years.

And I discovered that I had not written about my partner's Lyme disease once. I realized that anything that was causing me stress was of my own doing.

As a sidenote, one way to relieve any stress you may have is by journaling. Take fifteen minutes at the beginning or end of each day and just do a brain dump on your thoughts at that moment.

Don't be shy, and don't be afraid to hold back. The only one who will read the journals one day will be you.

Some Things You May Need to Do for Yourself

Loving someone who is a chronic Lyme survivor can be stressful. No one likes to see someone they love struggle, especially when you cannot do anything to help.

You may find yourself angry at not being able to do more, or because they don't seem to be getting any better, even with all they are doing to treat themselves. Many Lyme survivors I spoke with said that no one could feel what they were going through unless they had the disease, and of course, no one wants anyone they love to have it.

Here are some ideas of things to do for yourself:

- Create a charitable organization devoted to Lyme support.
- Do more fun things with your partner.
- Do more service activities.
- Exercise.
- Get more involved with your children's sports teams or hobbies.
- Get psychological counseling.
- Journal.
- Practice meditation.
- Read up on Lyme.

- Speak with other family members and friends about Lyme and what your chronic Lyme survivor might be going through.
- Speak with other partners or family members.
- Speak with your clergy.
- Start a podcast.
- Write a book.

But don't give up.

You love her.

Keep giving her the support she needs from you.

In the next chapter, I share social media sites that helped me understand the disease and what chronic Lyme survivors go through each day.

CHAPTER TEN
Facebook Helped Me—It Might Help You

Questions to Ponder:
- *What internet resources are available to you?*
- *What are Lyme survivors discussing among themselves?*
- *How would they suggest you support your partner?*
- *What can you do to learn more about Lyme?*

As I said before, prior to the summer of 2021, I had never read a book about Lyme. I had searched Lyme a few times, mainly to understand gluten allergies, but nothing more than that.

At the Institute for Excellence in Sales, a big part of what we do is connect sales authors, speakers, and experts with sales leaders at companies. I read almost everything published on sales or business development and still love to read hardcover books.

My reading list changed radically after searching "Lyme" on Amazon. A few dozen books came up, and I purchased and read them all. I looked for the books with the most reviews first, and then searched for other topics such as anxiety, women's illness, and chronic illness.

Soon, I got to know my Amazon Prime delivery person's first name.

I stacked the books on my bed and started reading. See Appendix A for a list of the books I recommend.

What I Learned on Facebook Groups

Another good way to learn about Lyme disease is by joining the Lyme disease groups on Facebook, even for a short time. I learned so much about Lyme disease in the groups and met many wonderful people.

Spending time in the Lyme Disease groups on Facebook, I learned what Lyme survivors go through each day. I was surprised to hear about the lack of support many people received from their partners or family members.

Every day, there would be two to three new posts from people whose partners, friends, and family had abandoned them. And then fifty other survivors would chime in about how they were or were not supported.

That was one of the reasons that prompted me to write this book. The lack of support many Lyme survivors get from family and friends was astounding.

Here's a typical question I saw posted in some of the comments:

Question: *"After falling ill with Lyme, how many of you were abandoned by your husband? How many survived thanks to his support and love?"*

"My now ex-boyfriend abandoned me."

"My husband supports me fully."

"I don't think I would have made it through without my husband. He was the best support system and partner. I'm forever grateful to him."

"Both family and my long-term friends turned their back on me."

"I'm currently about to get a divorce. My husband has been calling me lazy for the last four years. I can't take it anymore."

"Embarrassed to say, we've been married over thirty years, but he never supported my seven years of on-and-off treatment—financially or emotionally. Instead, he had my kids believing it was all in my head, never came to one doctor visit, and ignored the fact that I was taking over thirty pills/supplements a day."

"I was abandoned by my husband emotionally; therefore, I divorced him."

"I shake a lot, and my ex said I made him seasick. He left my daughters and me after two years."

"Abandoned at first and accused of lying/faking to get drugs. However, after six years and me beginning the process of moving out, he is now supportive."

"It would have been nice to have the love and support in the beginning, as I desperately needed it. But this is an invisible disease, and when you have doctor after doctor after doctor saying there's nothing wrong with you, it's hard for someone to believe that there is something wrong with you."

Helping Each Other

I learned that many in the Lyme community were suffering, but many were also full of hope.

I discovered a community of people that wants to help and support each other. It's so challenging to get proper medical care and answers, they rely on each other to advise on many things, including:

- Emotional support when things are not going well
- How to be supported
- How to treat symptoms
- What foods to eat and which to avoid
- How to interpret Lyme disease test results
- Which Lyme-literate medical doctors (LLMDs) to contact and how best to prepare for appointments
- Which protocols to follow
- Why certain things happen at certain times
- Why they might be experiencing certain things

And many more.

I witnessed overwhelming support every time someone asked a particular treatment question.

After pouring through endless books and learning new information, I wanted to know some of the ways people were treating themselves and how I could be more supportive. I learned about many herbal protocols and treatments that I did not know of before this journey.

I posted in one of the groups asking what questions a partner should ask to understand and be supportive.

This was a beneficial process in realizing how little support some Lyme survivors got from their family, partners, and friends.

Here's a sampling of the responses I received that day. It was overwhelming and gave an appreciation for the Lyme community's struggles. But it also gave me an appreciation for how just a little caring can go a long way.

It's also an excellent way to understand some things you can do to make your loved one's life a little easier.

I posted the question: *What questions should a partner ask to understand and be supportive?*

The answers fell into three categories:

1. Get Smarter—Many Lyme survivors who answered my question said they wished their partners or family members would become more conversant on the disease. They were constantly searching for answers and desired to see interest from those around them. Take a little bit of time and research beyond reading this book.
2. Ways to Help Show You Care
3. Understanding the Disease

Get Smarter

"Sounds SO familiar! Lymedisease.org has a wealth of information. Honestly, depending on how the infection affects her, questions can be hard to answer. There is so much happening that it's confusing even for the patient."

"Learn what you can from the research, be WITH her, and make sure she's getting all the medical support she should from a good Lyme clinic."

"My boyfriend once overheard me discussing my symptoms with a friend that I hadn't shared with him. He later asked me why I never told him, and I said because I didn't want to come across like I was complaining all the time. Because, truthfully, I could complain all the time. But he then said something that really touched me. He asked me to please share all my symptoms with him to be more aware of what I'm going through and that he would never mistake it for complaining."

"Just ask her to tell you more about her illness/history and feelings about it. Then she can tell you what she wants, and you can just listen and validate her feelings. Asking too many questions may seem controlling. Later, you might ask about which coinfections she has, which treatments she would like to do, or how you could help her."

"Asking what it's like to have Lyme could be good. And perhaps how can I support you, and how can I help you get the most out of life?"

Ways to Show You Care

"He helped me fold all the bedsheets/blankets due to my recent hand joint pain. [He also asks if he can] carry the heavy laundry hampers upstairs when done folding them so that I can put the clothes away, or [if he can] carry our daughter's monthly medical shipment boxes, which are heavy boxes (about ten), so that I could open them all and unload them in their storage bins. Also, I ask that he carry those heavy bins into the storage unit. I used to do these things myself for years, but now I've learned to be more careful with my body."

"Offering to bathe our daughter or push her in her stroller for some fresh air would be amazing when my legs hurt too much, etc. It's so much pressure and guilt on me, always making sure she's being taken care of, that it hurts to care for her. She is aggressive at times, and it's hard caring for her in general. Just start helping her when she's doing something around the house, especially when she complains about pain or fatigue."

"I have a hard time asking for help with my chores because he works full time (I don't work), and he cooks as well, because it's always been his preference. So he is just swamped helping in those ways. But as I'm getting older—forty-two now and just got diagnosed with chronic Lyme four months ago—I've learned to ask for help in ways where I know I wouldn't feel too guilty or inadequate if he does it on his own."

"Offer to help do some chores she typically does when parts of her body don't feel great. For example, I loved it when my hubby offered help folding our massive, never-ending laundry. However, I'd like it if he offered to help me do those things and not do them for me, as I'd prefer teamwork together. Or just offer to do it if I'm not feeling capable or have the time."

"Ask what can I do to help you feel a little better today? I think of pain like currency. You may want to know if she wants to spend time on something she enjoys and what enjoyable thing she would like to do."

"I think it's important to be flexible and remember that symptoms sometimes fluctuate hour to hour, day to day, or year to year. What works today may not help tomorrow."

"Over the years, I asked for help and articulated what I needed. However, I was failed by family and doctors and friends so often. A lot of people are unable or unwilling to provide that for me."

"You might ask if that resonates for her and if some trauma work like EMDR (eye movement desensitization and reprocessing) might help her also. It's been huge for me on my healing journey."

"Interestingly enough, I read another post on Facebook this morning about how hard it is for those dealing with trauma, which Lyme disease is, to ask for/trust help because we build walls when we can't find the support we need. She may also be struggling with knowing how to accept the support you offer. I know I have that issue."

"I am not understood or supported by my partner and have been told they resent me for being sick and not being able to work anymore. That's an excellent example of what NOT to say. It's a rough road for the chronically ill person and their partner, so be gentle with each other."

"Just simply ask, what do I need to know, what can I do for you, do you need anything from me, what can I do to make your life easier. It's hard having a chronic illness; most partners don't understand or want to understand (ex: I've been told you already had treatment)."

"One of the main issues I deal with is the need for emotional support. My husband has learned to ask when I need him to cheer me up and when I need him to empathize and mourn with me. Because his knee-jerk reaction when I am having a hard time is to tell me everything will be all right. Sometimes I really need to hear that everything will be all right, and then I don't need to control it or panic about it. But sometimes I need him to be sad with me for a minute."

"I have Lyme and here is what helps me feel supported: when my husband pours me a detox bath (two cups Epsom salt, a few drops lavender oil, and temperature very hot). When my husband creates a healing environment—essential oils in the diffuser, heated blanket warmed up, 'spa'-type music on Spotify—and pours me a cup of elixir tea. This makes me feel taken care of and brings me relief from my symptoms."

"I don't love being asked how I am all of the time even though my husband means well. It can be discouraging to say I don't feel good constantly. I asked him to change it to 'How is your body today?' because sometimes I'm awesome, but my body feels like crap. This helps me separate the two, so I don't feel like my life is always crappy."

Understanding the Disease

"Sometimes you need to listen to venting and provide feedback or help solve the problem. Knowing the difference (asking upfront) can make communication smoother."

"Also, great gift ideas for her would be gift certificates for massage, like lymphatic massage. I hear it helps with detox."

"Let her know it's okay to be honest about how much pain she is in."

"Look out for her 'sucking it up' or 'I'll push through' phrases that mean 'I am extending myself further than I should because I don't want to fail or take too long or be a burden or complain or not finish what we set out to do.'"

"The thing about this illness is it can be so isolating. You can feel very alone, even with a sea of people around you. It's a hard illness. I just want someone to say to me, 'I see you. I see how hard this is for you. I am here, and I will stand next to you every step of the way.' People don't need solutions; most of the time, they can work them out themselves. They want to feel recognized and understood."

"What didn't help with the symptoms? Can I help research any vitamins, supplements, or protocols you want to try? I keep a journal of meds, protocols, supplements, etc., so it's easier to look back and see everything written down. 'Lyme Brain/Brain Fog' is a real issue for many of us, so writing things down is a must. I also take my journal with me to any doctor appointments and ask the person who's with me to take notes for me."

"Ask her what it is like for her. What does a good day feel like? What does a bad day feel like?"

"Many of us have learned to try and do everything for ourselves, but what seem like daily tasks to others are more like running a marathon. Taking a shower, getting dressed, cooking a meal, any housework, etc., is exhausting. To have help with the little things can have a big impact on pain and energy levels. It's also very important to have emotional support. Feelings of guilt or shame, depression, and anxiety are very common in the Lyme community."

There are so many ways to support your partner or family member. Start by letting them know you love them and are there for them.

In the next chapter, we'll talk about nutrition and how Lyme disease impacts what you can and should not eat.

CHAPTER ELEVEN
Being Gluten-Free Before It Was Cool

Questions to Ponder:
- *Why is a gluten-free diet important to Lyme Survivors?*
- *Should you modify your diet to support your partner?*
- *How important is proper nutrition for Lyme treatment?*
- *Why is your partner concerned about a leaky gut?*

Nutrition plays a crucial role in the Lyme survivor's life. Adapting to a new eating lifestyle and knowing what to eat is perhaps the most crucial component of healing this disease. Supporting your loved one in dietary changes will be an adjustment. Hopefully, you can be flexible, patient, and take time together to create a list of foods to eat and not to eat.

I discovered that many Lyme survivors are gluten-free. Many have been gluten-free before gluten-free was the cool thing. Many Lyme-literate medical doctors (LLMDs) prescribe a gluten-free diet for Lyme survivors because gluten promotes inflammation in the body.

A person can be allergic to gluten and/or have a sensitivity to it. If allergic, they cannot have any cross-contamination of gluten. It is crucial to read labels on products and make sure they were made in a facility dedicated to gluten-free products.

Also, many people with Lyme cannot eat out at restaurants. There are too many cross-contaminants in restaurant food and in the kitchens. Even though a restaurant may say the food is gluten-free, you cannot be certain without dedicated spaces.

No one knew what gluten-free meant when we first started dating. We had to educate our friends and family on what gluten-free entailed. When we visited anyone, they supported getting gluten-free food to make it easier.

Going out to eat can be challenging. However, as gluten-free becomes more widely accepted, menu choices have expanded. Still, you may find that the only options are a piece of chicken or a hamburger without a bun and some veggies. If you want dessert after the meal, most likely the only option is a scoop of ice cream.

One thing that I got good at was finding the best gluten-free pizza wherever we went. Thank goodness for Yelp. We probably tried every brown rice flour, amaranth flour, buckwheat flour, chickpea flour, almond flour, cornmeal flour, millet flour, navy bean flour, quinoa flour, and cauliflower pizza crust known to humankind.

We explored every place that sold gluten-free pizza in the tri-state area. I did not mind shifting to gluten-free pizza, although there were times when I missed good old traditional pizza; however, my figure didn't.

Of course, due to the gluten allergy, your partner or family member might also need to refrain from drinking beer or brown liquors. Alcohol is an inflammatory food and should be avoided.

Alcohol can contribute to chronic inflammation. In fact, chronic inflammation is often linked to alcohol-related health conditions.

When your body metabolizes alcohol in your gastrointestinal (GI) tract, it can disrupt tissue homeostasis. This can cause a chronic state of inflammation in the intestines. Alcohol can also cause inflammation in the joints.

AnnaMarie Houlis states in her article "Alcohol and Inflammation" that "Because alcohol can cause inflammation, it can also be the root cause of joint and muscle pain. Alcohol intake can bring on or trigger existing joint and muscle pain." (Houlis 2022).

According to the Natural Paleo Family website, "Lyme can directly affect the liver, overburdening it with filtering out toxins excreted by the pathogens in your body. The result is that the excess toxins put it into a weakened state. Once in this weakened state, drinking alcohol can make it worse. The bottom line is that the body sees alcohol as poison, and when you drink it, the liver prioritizes the processing of the alcohol, and everything else gets put on hold in the meantime." (Natural Paleo Family 2020)

Blood sugar can get low when you have Lyme disease and coinfections. On one of our first dates, my partner and I drove near Atlantic City, heading to a local diner for dinner. My partner's blood sugar was running low. Luckily, I had some nut bars in the trunk.

According to Thomas Ball, when dealing with Lyme disease, what you eat is essential to your health. In addition to gluten, other foods to consider eliminating due to their inflammatory properties are sugar, dairy, legumes, soy, red meats, and more. (Ball 2020)

I read several articles that said to eat foods that provide a more alkaline environment than acidic. Supposedly Lyme bacteria cannot survive in a more alkaline environment.

What Is a Leaky Gut?

Finally, there is the whole leaky gut problem. Certain foods can cause the lining of the small intestine to weaken. As a result, small holes can develop that allow food particles and bad bacteria to escape the intestine into the bloodstream. If this happens, your immune system goes into attack mode, thus causing more inflammation.

Having a healthy small intestine is essential to absorb your vitamins and minerals.

Dairy and sugar may also need to be removed or at least limited from the diet. These products tend to have yeast, which promotes the growth of the bacteria. Animal's milk contains casein, a protein that can cause inflammation in the infected victims, according to drprem.com. (Global Health Care, n.d.)

Eliminating sugar is a priority. All these dietary components play a significant role in treating Lyme disease.

In a previous chapter, I introduced you to J. P. Davitt. He recommends an elimination diet to remove toxic ingredients from your daily intake. Specific foods to eliminate include:

- **Corn syrup**, which is addictive and causes the pancreas to use a massive amount of insulin. Pancreas health and insulin production is directly correlated to aging.

- **Hydrogenated oils** such as canola oil, which is another name for rapeseed oil. These oils are literally burnt, and the process that creates them builds toxicity in the body that destroys your hormones. In addition, these oils have a screwed-up molecular structure. They are found in margarine, fried foods, coffee creamers, potato chips, and packaged snacks.
- **Gluten**, which is in many foods because we cut corners and shortcut the manufacturing of our food. It causes holes in the intestines and leaks, causing autoimmune symptoms. (Davitt 2021)

Maintaining the best diet can be confusing. We will make mistakes, so making more good choices than bad sounds like our best option.

Although everyone has a different makeup, some anti-inflammatory foods that might help with recovery include:

- Avocado
- Coconut oil
- Fruits
- Leafy greens
- Nuts

In the next chapter, we'll discuss the six stages of healing.

CHAPTER TWELVE
The Six Stages of Healing

Questions to Ponder:
- *How do you help your partner heal?*
- *What do you need to heal from?*
- *What are the six stages of healing?*

If you're healthy, "healing" is probably a word you do not think about often. I never did but know that your Lyme survivor thinks about it every day.

When you love and care about someone, supporting them through their healing journey greatly benefits their progress. In *The Gratitude Curve*, Gregg Kirk has given a lot of thought to the healing process, which he says has six steps:

1. Discovery
2. Disillusionment
3. Treatment
4. Anger and Panic
5. Acceptance
6. Gratitude

One of the first books I read during my education of Lyme was his. He describes the pain he endured and his lengths to understand how to heal from his chronic Lyme. As mentioned earlier, Kirk also appeared on my podcast about discovering his life's mission after conquering Lyme.

We discussed his healing process in depth. The following does not apply to every chronic Lyme survivor. Some may get stuck in the process and find the order slightly different. Not everyone will get to the final stage either.

Kirk has published some of this information in various forms in the past. He has permitted me to repurpose it in this book. He's also been a source of information on Lyme for me and has done a fantastic job of giving back to the Lyme community with the Ticked Off Foundation.

Gregg's article, "The Six Stages to Chronic Lyme Healing," is posted as a blog on his personal website, www.greggkirk.com. His direct words follow in *italics*.

STAGE ONE: Discovery

Patients can get stuck in this stage for months, years, and even decades. They know something is wrong with them, but they don't know exactly what. They go from doctor to doctor and take test after test and still don't reach an adequate explanation for the wide range of symptoms they're experiencing. Or worse, misdiagnosis may send them down a treatment rabbit hole with no end solution.

When a definitive diagnosis does come through, the patient feels an overwhelming sense of relief that they can now focus on their disease with a treatment that will ultimately bring them to complete recovery. For the chronic Lyme patient, this relief is short-lived, as they begin to experience the challenges of the Treatment phase.

STAGE TWO: Disillusionment

This stage may come during the Discover stage or the Treatment stage. Either way, a chronic Lyme patient will begin to have some of their beliefs about their trusted medical systems, insurance coverage, and Western medical doctors' knowledge overturned. Every chronic Lyme patient expects to go to a trusted physician, get a timely and accurate diagnosis, and begin an effective treatment protocol that eliminates the illness. This process helped them recover from colds, flu, and other acute illnesses, so why wouldn't this work for Lyme disease?

As the chronic Lyme patient begins to experience inconclusive or incorrect diagnoses and treatment protocols that are dangerous and ineffective in curing them, they lose faith in the system that had previously supported them. They find that insurance companies don't cover alternative treatments and barely cover pharmaceutical treatments that often don't help. If their doctors have not been trained in chronic Lyme treatment, these physicians can become defensive and question whether their patients are sick with a legitimate disease.

Family members may begin to believe that the chronic Lyme patient's illness is all in their head and that they are either seeking attention or suffering from depression or mental illness. At this point, the patient who can move from disillusionment through a belief-system shift of self-empowerment (by becoming their own health advocate or even their own physician) is the patient who can move up in the hierarchy.

STAGE THREE: Treatment

Treatment of chronic Lyme is not a one-size-fits-all proposition. Physicians and patients find that the treatment combinations that work effectively tend to be customized to the patient and their set of symptoms and coinfections. It is important that a patient goes through the Disillusionment phase by realizing that the scenario they experienced in the past of diagnosis/treatment/cure will not be the same straight line with chronic Lyme. Further confusing is that because antibiotics are prescribed and proven effective in treating early-onset Lyme, many physicians prescribe antibiotics-only treatments to their chronic Lyme patients.

These patients may experience some early symptom relief. Still, many cannot tolerate antibiotics alone or they find they need to continue treatment when their symptoms return weeks, months, or years later. Most physicians agree that while antibiotics-only treatment may give some relief, it is not a cure for chronic Lyme disease. The patients who reach complete healing move to all-natural and herbal remedies to remove the pathogens with a combination of detoxifiers that eliminate toxins from their system without suffering from endless Herxheimer reactions.

At this point, it can be an important move for a patient to do their own research and find the treatment combinations that work for them. This move to self-empowerment can help guide them through the later stages of healing.

STAGE FOUR: Anger and Panic

For those stuck in the Disillusionment and/or Treatment stages, overwhelming frustration with lack of healing improvement can bring up combinations of anger, rage, and panic in chronic Lyme patients.

Depending on the patient, they can react either externally or internally, which can have a bearing on whether the patient experiences anger or panic. Patients who react externally are more prone to anger and tend to get frustrated with their family members, doctors, and support systems. They can flare into rages that alienate them from the very people trying to help them.

Further, they can feel unheard or marginalized when they complain of symptoms and don't receive validation from others. Because these patients tend to suffer from central nervous system irritation brought on by Bartonella and other coinfections, the term "Bartonella Rage" has become well-known in chronic Lyme communities.

If a patient reacts internally, they may be prone to fits of panic. It is common for Lyme patients to run out of money and support during the treatment stage, and these stressors can result in the patient feeling hopeless. When the bottom falls out of a patient's world like this, and they have no energy to continue fighting the illness, suicidal thoughts occur. It is unfortunate that suicide continues to be the leading cause of death in Lyme patients in the United States.

This stage may also seem like you're playing "Whack a Mole." You take care of one thing, and then another symptom appears.

For these reasons, patients need to move beyond this stage. Furthermore, the anger and panic they experience worsen symptoms and help the bacteria and coinfections thrive. Those who have come to terms with their anger and panic find they have more energy reserves to heal. They focus on moving on with their lives versus feeling the need to prove the injustices they have experienced.

To be sure, they have suffered real injustices, but it is exhausting and energy-draining to spend your time proving yourself to an unsympathetic audience. Placing focus on happier thoughts, successes, and positive pursuits has always proven to be a powerful component to healing, and it is the key to helping patients move on from this stage.

STAGE FIVE: Acceptance

A patient who has accepted his/her situation is ripe for healing. It doesn't mean they have resigned themselves to failure. It means they have stopped resisting and have stopped the energy cycle of opposing force from the disease.

Many alternative healers will tell you the less energy and attention you give to an illness, the less resistance you will get back from it. I noticed this during my own healing journey. The more I focused on the symptoms and bad feelings the disease was causing, the worse I felt. Yet, there were times when I would watch a funny show on TV or listen to some music that made me forget I was sick. The more I strung those situations together into longer periods of time, the better and better I felt.

Another way to let go of resistance during this stage is to stop identifying with the illness. Stop calling it "my disease" or "my symptoms." The bottom line and the best way to move through this stage is to accept the illness while also stopping the amount of energy and attention you give it. Once negative focus on the illness has dwindled to almost nothing, patients tend to move to the next stage.

STAGE SIX: Gratitude

If the idea of being grateful for chronic Lyme disease coming into your life sounds ridiculous or unthinkable, you may not be ready for this stage. Those who have reached recovery openly accept this concept. It allows them to put the illness completely behind them and understand why it was introduced in their life in the first place. It helps to think of the disease as simply new information introduced into one's life.

The illness is a doorway or fork in the road that can either take you upwards or downwards. Instead of reacting negatively, you can accept it gracefully and realize what a gift of experience you were given. This experience can be like a forest fire that burns away all unnecessary elements in your life while creating space for new growth. Yes, it burns things you deem valuable, but after those things are gone, you realize they weren't as important as you thought.

(The Gratitude Curve 2017)

Help your Lyme survivor get to Stage Six, Gratitude.

Your Lyme survivor didn't ask for this disease, nor did you. Be patient and understanding if it takes time to meet these stages. You may feel like giving up, which is normal, but you are stronger getting through this together. At the Acceptance stage, your partner can understand how much you love her and how much you mean to her. Love, not need or desire, happens at this stage. It's a powerful place to arrive at.

In the next chapter, we'll discuss why it's so expensive to treat Lyme disease.

CHAPTER THIRTEEN
Politics, Expense, Insurance

Questions to Ponder:
- *Why is it so expensive to treat Lyme?*
- *Why doesn't insurance cover chronic Lyme?*
- *Why does the CDC contend that chronic Lyme even exists?*

I was shocked to learn three things about Lyme medical treatment:
- Since so few doctors know how to treat Lyme, it's another reason why Lyme-literate medical doctor (LLMD) care comes at a premium.
- Many people cannot get treatment since insurance does not typically cover Lyme treatment post thirty days of antibiotics.
- 99 percent of allopathic medical practitioners will not believe the patient is sick or that chronic Lyme even exists.

And you want to hear something crazy? The politics associated with this disease will impact you and your partner's quality of life!

As mentioned previously, some official entities, such as the CDC, dispute whether chronic Lyme exists!

Is your partner or family member in pain, riddled by anxiety, spending all their time trying to heal? If so, I'd say that something exists!

Dr. Richard Horowitz, the author of one of the books I reference in Appendix A, said in an article on LymeDisease.org in January 2017:

> The symptoms of tick-borne illness often mimic those of other commonly reported diseases that are diagnosed based on clinical criteria and not definitive laboratory testing. These include fibromyalgia, chronic fatigue syndrome (Systemic Exertional Intolerance Disease), multiple sclerosis, mental illness, and many others. These figures would not be included in the statistics of those affected.

> The Infectious Disease Society of America (IDSA) calls these patient complaints and reported suffering "post-Lyme disease treatment syndrome" and makes the assumption that patients' continuing symptoms of fatigue, joint/muscle pain, and cognitive dysfunction are not the result of persistent, active infection.
>
> Other clinicians believe that persistence of Lyme and other tick-borne diseases are due to chronic infection and that chronic Borreliosis and associated tick-borne infections might be putting future generations at risk through maternal-fetal transmission and contaminated blood supplies. (Horowitz 2017)

Listen. I'm not a political person, and I'm not a conspiracy theorist, but when you break an ankle, everyone agrees that you broke an ankle.

Not everyone agrees that this disease even exists! And this is going to cause you a lot of emotional and financial distress.

I had a conversation with a relative who has a close friend who is an infectious disease doctor. When my relative told the doctor about Lyme symptoms, the friend said, "Well, you know that chronic Lyme doesn't exist, right?"

Now, not to split hairs, but I know someone who's in pain when I see them, and you probably do as well. And while the infectious disease community may have a point (if the bacteria is gone, then there's no lingering infectious disease), your partner is still fatigued, in pain, anxious, and miserable. Unfortunately, no test can prove the infection is completely gone.

And that, my friend, is going to affect your life.

My discovery of how politics, expenses, and insurance played a role in Lyme disease treatment was quite shocking. Unfortunately, many Lyme survivors go through years of being misdiagnosed. Of course, the longer it takes to get properly diagnosed, the less chance of effectively eradicating the disease from the body.

Some people get bitten, later have fatigue, pain, or other symptoms, and then go through years of being improperly diagnosed. If you live in Connecticut, where Lyme is commonly known, you might get diagnosed quicker, but if you live where not many doctors or other medical practitioners are aware of Lyme, it can easily be misdiagnosed.

And family members might dispute that they are sick, which does not help matters. They may have symptoms, then google, "Does chronic

Lyme exist?" only to see information posted by the CDC or IDSA, so then they deny they even have something.

And there are chronic Lyme survivors who test positive even by the CDC standards!

A common scenario can be:

- A person gets bit.
- Symptoms start.
- They go see a doctor who is not trained to detect Lyme disease and is thus unable to detect the problem. If the blood work is clean, it's not uncommon for the patient to be told it's all in their head.

Many people do not even know they were bitten by a tick. They never see the "bullseye rash," which is a common sign that a tick bite happened. The nymphal ticks are so small, and the larvae are smaller (they carry *Borrelia miyamotoi*, which is another tick-borne disease). People who are bitten may not see a tick and may never get a rash.

There are so many scenarios as to why people do not get diagnosed properly, which is why a tick-borne disease specialist is so important. MDs usually do not want to treat Lyme, as they cannot take insurance since insurance companies will limit the length of time and type of treatment. They also get investigated by medical licensing boards. So if they only take private payment, they can avoid being on the radar somewhat.

An LLMD would look for signs, symptoms, and history, and would rule out other medical conditions. They use testing as supportive care. Also, they look for coinfections, and as we've mentioned previously, most Lyme survivors have them.

The mystery illness.

It can be very frustrating. It might take years, sometimes decades, to get properly diagnosed. And, of course, at that point, your partner might have suffered through years of torment, pain, and fatigue.

It can be frustrating. You may wonder, why are they always sick? Why don't they have energy? Why are they sleeping so much?

Here's something to know: **It bothers them more than you!**

Cost of Treatment

Lyme treatment can vary, mainly because there is no standard treatment. We've discussed antibiotics and herbals, but the range of treatment is broad, especially if an ill-informed doctor is treating only symptoms.

And this can go on for decades.

Listen, you do not need to go to Washington, DC, or spend all your time on the internet understanding the bureaucracy behind the resistance to determine if chronic Lyme even exists. You need to know, though, that it is a quagmire, within a conundrum, wrapped in a puzzle. And it's going to cost you a lot of money.

As I mentioned, there are debates throughout the bureaucratic agencies about whether this disease even exists.

The problem for you, the partner, is that if these debates go on, costs to treat your loved one will continue to be absurdly high, and you're probably going to struggle to afford them.

[NOTE: There are some charities that offer small gifts to cover medicine and other treatment. Seek them out online or in your community.]

That's going to cause a financial burden and make things even more challenging. You'll want to spend all your money on treating the disease because that's what loving couples do for each other.

But that means you may not go on vacations, your discretionary funds may go to treatment, kids may not be able to go to the college of their choice, and friction may ensue.

And if your partner cannot work because of the effects of the disease, she may feel guilty and feel like a burden to you. [PS: Remind her that she isn't.]

The Tick-Borne Disease Working Group

According to the U.S. Department of Health and Human Services (HHS) website (hhs.gov), here's the mission of the Tick-Borne Disease Working Group:

"The Tick-Borne Disease Working Group (TBDWG) was established by Congress in 2016 as part of the 21st Century Cures Act to provide subject matter expertise and to review federal efforts related to all tick-borne diseases, to help ensure interagency coordination and minimize overlap, and to examine research priorities." (Health and Human Services 2020)

Again, the purpose of this book is not to get political. It's to help partners, family members, and friends of chronic Lyme survivors understand what their loved one is going through to provide the most loving support and prepare for what lies ahead.

But you should know about this in case you want to get involved with making your local legislature more aware of the epidemic that Lyme is. When I started writing blogs, people reached out to me to thank me for making more people aware of the disease.

Below are excerpts from written comments received by the TBDWG for its March 2020 meeting. You'll see how challenging this disease is for the community, let alone your partner, who is just trying to survive and make it through the day.

The complete record can be found on the hhs.gov website.

Here is the partial testimony of Lucy Barnes, a Lyme survivor for over 40 years.

(Barnes notes facts as listed by the Tick-Borne Disease Working Group of the Office of the Assistant Secretary for HHS.)

- As of March 2020, there is still no accurate test (74.9 percent of infected patients missed)
- Still no successful prevention methods (with over 1,500 published studies and billions spent)
- Still no successful treatments (that work broadly for most patients)

Recommendations by the IDSA and CDC consist of referrals to psychiatrists and OTC medications for devastating, ongoing, and worsening symptoms caused by an infectious disease.

The lack of a vaccine has caused billions of dollars to be spent on treatments that may or may not work.

Andrea Jackson, of Weld County, Colorado, testified:

The CDC and other federal agencies base their support of false "Lyme myths" on statistics contrived from testing now proven to give false negatives to 71 percent.... For decades, the CDC pushed doctors to not test unless in a state labeled as "high incident states" and required that if they did test, they must use the 71 percent-false-negative test. ALL the Lyme statistics used to push Lyme myths have been based on this failed testing. The TBDWG agencies reps refuse to re-educate the doctors and public that they have ensured [who] believe: Lyme is rare and easy to cure, only occurs in a few areas, does not exist in a persistent form, can't be passed from mother to child or between partners, and does not require long-term antibiotics to address in its persistent form.

Lyme disease is NOT rare and easy to cure!

A Challenge for Treatment

There are two camps. Let's start with the CDC and the IDSA. The IDSA enforces the CDC standards in partnership with the insurance industry.

Many people ask why Lyme disease is not covered by medical insurance and why their LLMD does not take insurance. The IDSA advocates for the CDC company line of thirty days of doxycycline for adults and thirty days of amoxycillin for kids.

If you have any Lyme disease symptoms post the thirty-one days, IDSA says you have Post Treatment Lyme Disease Syndrome (PTLDS). Based on this position, some doctors would be inferring that the Lyme survivor is exaggerating the symptoms. Others will say it's like nerve damage and you don't have an infection anymore.

There's the dilemma.

And why is this a continuing problem for you?

It's not about science. It comes down to what's known as "regulatory capture." An economic theory determines why you cannot pay for a doctor, why insurance does not cover chronic Lyme, and why your life is miserable.

According to the financial website Investopedia, "Regulatory capture is an economic theory that says regulatory agencies may come to be dominated by the industries or interests they are charged with regulating. The result is that an agency, charged with acting in the public interest, instead acts in ways that benefit incumbent firms in the industry it is supposed to be regulating." (Investopedia 2021)

It means that participants in the industry, usually larger enterprises with deep financial interests, tend to fight for their interests versus individuals or those with less lobbying power. In other words, the insurance companies don't want to pay for your ongoing treatment for a disease that the government agency says doesn't even exist! As a result, the insurance lobby firms are much more powerful than the individual Lyme patients or the few entities that advocate for your partner.

And because of that, your medical insurance will not cover your treatment beyond the thirty days of antibiotics. Treatment is not driven by science. It's driven by insurance and medical association influence.

Now I have heard that you possibly can get insurance to cover Lyme treatment past thirty days. Still, it may require litigation, and the insurance company will often settle right before a trial or summary judgment and pay for the treatment. Most Lyme survivors do not have the time, energy, or resources to pursue this path. I've heard of some cases where the insurance company settled right before trial began. This is so there would be no "case law" of any type on the record in any court.

The insurance companies do not want to pay for long-term IV antibiotic therapy costing hundreds of thousands of dollars per year. Some of the treatments your partner may want to consider are not conventional ones, and insurance companies do not typically cover alternative treatments.

By the way, the fifty state medical boards are also involved with regulatory capture. It's a giant spider web of groupthink, the establishment, corruption, and status quo.

And you and your partner are caught in this web. She has a disease affecting her body, mind, and soul, while the regulatory agencies can go to sleep at night knowing that they are covered.

The costs of treating this disease are something you probably have not budgeted to spend. Make sure you have a plan in place to pay for treatment. It won't be easy but getting ahead of the curve will help you down the road.

In the next chapter, we'll discuss why you're going to be doing most of this on your own.

CHAPTER FOURTEEN
Becoming Your Own Health Care Advocate

Questions to Ponder:
- *Why is your partner consumed with her Lyme symptoms?*
- *How can you be supportive and understand the symptoms?*
- *Why does she know more than the doctors?*

I've learned that many Lyme survivors feel alone with their illness and symptoms. They often feel clueless and live in a world of uncertainty, not knowing why certain symptoms occur or how they will feel each day. Then, when they go to a doctor, they may feel even more alone and frustrated that the doctor has limited knowledge of Lyme treatment.

The doctor will try to help, but the wrong treatment may be prescribed, which won't help and could possibly be harmful. I've heard from many Lyme survivors that their doctors have misdiagnosed the Lyme as fibromyalgia, chronic fatigue syndrome (CFS), MS, a neuropsychiatric disorder, or, unfortunately, a psychosomatic disorder.

Also unfortunately, the Lyme survivor may not be properly diagnosed for years until they see a doctor who is knowledgeable about Lyme disease.

If the underlying problem is a tick-borne illness, it may go undiagnosed, and thus be incorrectly treated for years and perhaps decades.

You and your Lyme survivor may leave doctor appointments feeling they were a waste of time and money, and you may refuse to seek additional help. Now the research to understand the disease inside and out and become your own health advocate begins. It will be a challenge to figure everything out.

She's sick with something she does not even know that she has.

And it will linger.

And it will fester.

Since she cannot figure out what she has, it's not uncommon for your partner to become a medical detective.

As she tries to determine why she's experiencing specific symptoms, she may spend hours on the internet researching and seeking possible solutions.

Eventually, she will know more about how the disease and the treatments will affect her than her doctor does, even if the doctor is a top Lyme-literate medical doctor (LLMD). Also, many doctors have a cookie-cutter treatment for all patients. The treatments are not tailored for each unique individual and their symptoms, no matter what their specific symptoms might be. She may feel she's already been there and done that.

Be supportive with what she eats, her sleep patterns, and how the environment impacts their health.

Give her space to heal as well.

Believe and Stand Up for Them

Unfortunately, too many people, friends, and family members think Lyme is "fake" and are lying about being ill. It is easy to dismiss a disease that you cannot see. It is important to remember to be a partner and a team to fight Lyme together. To support them means believing in them even if you don't understand everything 100 percent. It means standing up for them when others don't.

This schism in the medical community can have massive impacts on spousal and family support (both socially and financially). Unfortunately, what happens with many partners and family members is that, for those who believe what they read on the internet, it often leads to abuse of the Lyme patient, who gets labeled a "faker," "attention seeker," "psych patient," or worse.

And then, the abuse often gets taken a step further. I've heard of some partners or family members who have tried to get the Lyme patient institutionalized. This is also accompanied in some families by emotional, verbal, and sometimes physical abuse.

The CDC Discourages the Term "Chronic Lyme"

Part of the challenges faced is the confusion spread by the CDC about if *chronic Lyme* even exists. The CDC disputes that it does and prefers the term Post Treatment Lyme Disease Syndrome (PTLDS).

The problem is, what if your partner was infected years ago but was never treated for Lyme? I've met many people who never recall getting bitten and then suffer for years or decades before receiving any type of treatment. This leads to the disrespect they may get from family and medical professionals.

Here's how it's described on the CDC website:

> Lyme disease is caused by infection with the bacterium *Borrelia burgdorferi*. Although most cases of Lyme disease can be cured with a 2- to 4-week course of oral antibiotics, patients can sometimes have symptoms of pain, fatigue, or difficulty thinking that lasts for more than 6 months after they finish treatment. This condition is called Post-Treatment Lyme Disease Syndrome (PTLDS).
>
> Why some patients experience PTLDS is not known. Some experts believe that *Borrelia burgdorferi* can trigger an "autoimmune" response causing symptoms that last well after the infection itself is gone. Autoimmune responses are known to occur following other infections, including campylobacter (Guillain-Barré syndrome), chlamydia (Reiter's syndrome), and strep throat (rheumatic heart disease). Other experts hypothesize that PTLDS results from a persistent but difficult to detect infection. Finally, some believe that the symptoms of PTLDS are due to other causes unrelated to the patient's *Borrelia burgdorferi* infection.
>
> Unfortunately, there is no proven treatment for PTLDS. Although short-term antibiotic treatment is a proven treatment for early Lyme disease, studies funded by the National Institutes of Health (NIH) have found that long-term outcomes are no better for patients who received additional prolonged antibiotic treatment than for patients who received placebo. Long-term antibiotic treatment for Lyme disease has been associated with serious, sometimes deadly complications, as described in the links below.
>
> Patients with PTLDS usually get better over time, but it can take many months to feel completely well. If you have been treated for

Lyme disease and still feel unwell, see your healthcare provider to discuss additional options for managing your symptoms. If you are considering long-term antibiotic treatment for ongoing symptoms associated with a Lyme disease infection, please talk to your healthcare provider about the possible risks of such treatment. (Centers for Disease Control 2022)

Treatment Options

Through my research and connecting with others, I learned important things for you to know about your Lyme disease survivor and her recovery.

As I've stated many times, Lyme disease is challenging to treat. However, many varied treatments can put it into remission and make life much more pleasant.

There are two general ways to treat the disease. First is the "Western medicine" antibiotic route. There is no standard antibiotic route, as most patients have coinfections, and each case is different. Getting antibiotics intravenously is a common approach.

The second treatment approach is from the "terrain theory," a term from the alternative medicine world. Alternative medicine does not have to be radical. Many cancer treatments, for example, are based on terrain theory.

In terrain theory, any infection is considered environmental, so you want to clean up all the possible environmental variables weakening your body. I spoke with a Lyme survivor who had his most significant breakthrough by getting more sunlight! He said he was outside for two hours and noticed that he was feeling much better. There were no other variables, and he had not taken anything else during that time.

While Lyme is typically an acute infection in its early stages, it morphs into a terrain disease. At this stage, the Lyme will tend to exacerbate any pre-existing physical deficiencies that a person has (or had), creating a vicious cycle where the Lyme gets worse, along with that physical deficiency.

For example, in people whose primary effects from Lyme are cardiac, those patients often had some history of a previous cardiac issue. Or some people might also have a parasite infection, which needs treatment to achieve higher odds of success. As a rule, the longer the time between the tick bite and the diagnosis, the more these "terrain factors" become barriers to healing, which must be addressed to maximize the odds of Lyme treatment success.

Biohacking and Crowdcuring

Another advance in recent years is what's known as biohacking. According to Darya Sinusoid, "biohacking refers to any practices aimed at enhancing your biology. Examples [include] having a simple healthy lifestyle like getting enough sleep and eating clean, to more radical practices like chip implants, cryotherapy, and neurofeedback." (Shortform, 2021)

Biohacking also looks back at a lot of the forgotten remedies. For example, when you study infectious disease treatment from 100 years ago, you see that during the pandemic in 1918, many people found that sunlight helped cure certain infections.

It's about connecting dots.

Crowdcuring is when the community comes together to help each other figure out ways to treat the illness. The advice is based on common experiences, and treatment successes and failures.

A lot of work is being done to understand mitochondrial biohacking. The mitochondria are the most important cells in your body. One of the most important fuels of the mitochondria is electrons. Lyme survivors need to rebuild their mitochondria and the efficiency of what's called the electron transport chain. There are many ways to do that.

For one thing, let's talk about sunlight a bit more. Sunlight gives you, for example, infrared light, UVA, and UVB, and those all improve health. This is because it improves the efficiency of the electron transport chain.

Another treatment option is magnetics. We all get some level of magnetism from the Earth, known as Schumann Resonance. The Schumann Resonance is a frequency. It's the measurement of 7.83 Hz or the electromagnetic frequency of our planet, to be exact.

Many cultures implement vibrational techniques to synchronize with the frequencies of the Schumann Resonance or the "heartbeat" of mother earth. They believe that these frequencies can heal the body and mind as energies connect. Even in the ebb and flow of these energies, reducing high blood pressure and depression is somehow alleviated.

To help combat Lyme disease, some people use a Schumann Resonance device such as a rife machine that destroys micro-organisms using frequencies. Each organism has a different frequency setting. The machine can be set to destroy whatever is operating at that frequency. And some people swear by this.

Patience

Remember that these treatments take time.

I'll see people ask for advice on the internet, and I'll see the response, "I tried that one weekend, and it didn't work."

No treatment will work over a weekend. But what also happens, and what becomes a confusing barrier for so many patients and their caregivers, is that valid treatments will often make a person feel worse before they feel better. This can be from a Herxheimer reaction, where dying pathogens release toxins, but it can also be from the general detoxification that occurs as the body repairs itself.

That latter process occurs because repair and regeneration are inflammatory processes. But more specifically, there is often a form of "refeeding syndrome" that occurs as the patient's body is replenished and heals. We see this, for example, in other conditions like beriberi, where people who start taking Vitamin B1 will often get much sicker before they get better.

Adding to all of that, what's even more frustrating for patients and caregivers is that some doctors do not even mention these risks from the healing process, let alone know how to advise patients on managing those risk symptoms.

One of the problems with Lyme is that survivors, such as your partner, can become desperate. You need to understand that you're in it for the long haul and need to help them be patient. If trying a new approach that the LLMD recommends, you need to trust that it might solve a problem, although not right away.

Patience is the key issue in conquering this disease and getting it into remission.

The reason being, when you want to try and kill an infection, think of it as a complex set of building blocks that you need to have in place. The analogy is that a chain is only as strong as its links, so if your links are in very bad shape, you're not going to have success.

It might take years to figure it out.

It's a complex process, and there's no magic bullet.

It is easy to become discouraged and to give up on finding a treatment that will help, because it seems it may consume the rest of your life.

Remember to take a breath and take it one step at a time, so it isn't overwhelming. Some people's perception of the medical system goes back to the doctors we went to as kids. Most of the time, when you go to the doctor, he prescribes a pill, and you're good, right? People have that mentality going into these complex chronic diseases, but it doesn't work that way.

Understand that and work together to be patient.

In the next chapter, we will discuss what Lyme survivors are talking about with each other.

CHAPTER FIFTEEN
What Lyme Survivors Ask Each Other

Questions to Ponder:
- *What is on your partner's mind that she's not telling you?*
- *What are Lyme survivors asking each other?*
- *Why is she consumed with her disease?*

Since there are so many variables in figuring out how to treat Lyme disease, many Lyme survivors often rely on each other for support and information. I mentioned earlier in the book how I learned so much on Facebook. I learned that there are so many questions that need answering.

To give you an idea of what your partner might be wondering about, check out the list below of more than thirty questions that were posted during six hours on one of the most popular Facebook groups for Lyme survivors.

1. Is anybody else suffering from extreme dizziness, vertigo, imbalance, and lightheadedness from Lyme?
2. Does anybody have pain in their skull and spine?
3. Does anyone else freak out reading about candida in the blood causing septic shock?
4. Anyone else's weakness spread, making different body parts shake, like with weakness?
5. Has anyone ever thought the reason we never get better, even though we see LLMD and pound down antibiotics and herbs, is because we may be treating the wrong infection?
6. *Babesiosis*—How long can it last?
7. What is the best and quickest remedy for vertigo?

8. Can anyone recommend a quality LLMD they've used or had success with?
9. Can brain inflammation from this cause brain damage?
10. Does anybody else get painful sores all over your scalp, and if so, what have you found that helps?
11. Does anybody else suffer from this AWFUL lower back pain?
12. Does anybody suffer neuralgia (nerve pain in the head and face), and does anything help it?
13. Does this look like a tick bite?
14. Epstein Barr and candida are very high for me, followed by Babesia markers. I would like to hear what has been most effective for treating EB and candida?
15. Ever feel like the words don't come out right?
16. Has anyone else been up for the last three days? The full moon is causing havoc for me.
17. Has anyone had hyperthermia treatment?
18. Has anyone tried a hyperbaric oxygen chamber for pain and/or Lyme?
19. How do we know if it's a Lyme flare-up or just our immune system is so suppressed that we often get sick?
20. How do you deal with primary care physicians who don't believe your Lyme diagnosis or are dismissive of treatment?
21. How important do you think diet is in recovering from Lyme?
22. How many weeks of doxycycline should I request?
23. I'm not sure how to proceed due to chronic Lyme and other things. I have histamine intolerance and MCAS (mast cell activation syndrome). Thus, anything fermented, and soy as well cause my skin to flare and break out in hives.
24. Is anxiety common with Lyme?
25. Is there a connection between autistic spectrum disorders and tick-borne illnesses?
26. Is there a connection between Lyme and endometriosis?
27. Other options that would work like the biofilm dissolver Natto Plus supplement?

28. What supplements/antibiotics/drugs can you take that work for treating Bartonella if you have MCAS?
29. Which prescription/supplement helps you with acute panic attacks?
30. Why do Lyme and mold go hand in hand?

Your head is probably pounding from seeing all these questions, but it gives you a little peek into what your partner is thinking.

Since Lyme produces so many symptoms, it is not uncommon for Lyme survivors to believe that everything that occurs is a Lyme symptom. When asking these questions, it's not unusual to see a string of "yes, yes, yes" answers displayed. You may also see a string of answers meaning these questions have been already answered by others.

Understand that your partner is trying to put together a giant puzzle with more and more pieces being revealed. If she asks for your help, be ready to help.

In the next chapter, we'll discuss why it's important to cherish the fun moments you've shared over the years.

CHAPTER SIXTEEN
Love, Cherish, and Laugh

Questions to Ponder:
- *Can you find any humor in this?*
- *What are some things to do to add laughter into your lives?*
- *How do you know what your partner expects and needs?*

Lyme disease is not funny.

If you do a Google search on "Lyme disease funny" hardly anything will appear.

Conversely, there are plenty of cancer comedians. Go to YouTube and search "cancer comedy," and many videos will appear. Search "Lyme comedians" and few will appear.

This does not mean that you cannot make each other laugh. We laughed all the time. My partner was very funny, and we watched comedy videos all the time. Ten o'clock was *Seinfeld* time.

The first cute line she had was when we visited my parents in Atlantic City. Where my parents lived was not very touristy, so there weren't the amusements she was used to when she vacationed in North Carolina. After dinner the first night we were there, she asked if we could play putt-putt. I said there was no putt-putt in the area.

She said, "If there's no putt-putt, what's there to do?"

I said, "I don't know. Go to the casino?"

One hot summer night, we went to see Joan Jett and Styx perform. It was the second year in a row we had seen Styx. Thirty minutes into the set, after Tommy Shaw said they were going to play something from their new album, she said, "If we leave now, we can get to Dairy Queen by ten."

Hilarious.

She had some other gems.

She once said she was feeling very depressed a while back. I said, "Oh, before you met me?" She said, "No, last week."

Ouch.

We were big music fans and went to a lot of concerts. We saw 38 Special open for George Thorogood. Both groups put on an amazing show. I said, "I didn't know you liked 38 Special so much."

She said, "I'm a huge fan. Huge!"

That became a catch phrase.

There was a quilting place near our house. For a school project, my daughter wanted to go there. When we got there, it was what you would expect in a quilting supply store. Very serene. Peaceful. Quiet.

My partner asked the owner, "Are there any cases of ax murderers slashing quilters?"

I thought the owner was going to have a heart attack.

We were once talking about where we wanted to live in the future.

I said how about a nice house in a valley. She snapped a Zee and said, "I will not live in a valley!"

We never moved to a valley.

Laugh together. Make her laugh. Bring joy to her life and yours.

You can do this.

I'll offer some final thoughts on how you both can get through this in the next chapter.

CHAPTER SEVENTEEN
Final Thoughts

No doubt, having someone you love in your life who has Lyme disease can be a challenge. It probably makes you sad to see someone you care about living with this mysterious disease.

But you can get through it together by being supportive and learning about Lyme disease together. Many chronic Lyme survivors have overcome the disease with the proper medical care.

You have an opportunity to build a deeper, loving relationship by understanding what your partner is experiencing. I am glad that I took the time to learn more about Lyme disease to understand what Lyme survivors go through and how little is known about it. This mysterious disease needs to be more well known.

I loved every second I spent with my partner. I was lucky that she enjoyed watching sports and was genuinely interested in the games. Every night, we would watch basketball, hockey, football, or baseball. I'm from Philadelphia, so I always got excited watching the Phillies when they came on.

We loved comedy, so we watched a lot of *Seinfeld* and binged *Curb Your Enthusiasm*. We referenced both all the time. *Law and Order*, too.

When you understand more about how Lyme disease afflicts one you love, it changes you and makes you question everything. It certainly did for me. My increased education on this disease and how it has affected so many people has caused me to question everything I believe in. My thoughts on the meaning and purpose of life have changed. I now try to live by Einstein's quote that "Only a life lived in the service to others is a life worth living."

Show your partner or loved one how much you care for and cherish them. Let them know that this disease does not define them, and that they still have a purpose—a purpose to make a difference in the world, and to be loved.

Thank you for reading *Love, Hope, Lyme*. I hope it helps to strengthen your relationship and helps you to understand what it is like to live in a world of tick-borne illness.

All because a few months, years, or decades ago, someone you love, through no fault of their own, was bitten by an insect.

Live well.

Laugh often.

Love much.

Where there is love, there is hope.

References

Ball, Thomas. 2020. "The Top 10 Inflammatory Foods to Avoid." Performance Health Center. https://performancehealthcenter.com/2020/02/the-top-10-inflammatory-foods-to-avoid/.

Centers for Disease Control. 2022. "Post-Treatment Lyme Disease Syndrome." https://www.cdc.gov/lyme/postlds/index.html.

Davitt, J. P. 2021. *Lymebook: A Journey to Becoming One Day Better.* Independently Published.

Davitt, J. P. "How These Leaders Discovered Their 'Why' After Conquering Chronic Illness and How It Applies to Sales." July 6, 2021, on *Sales Game Changers Podcast*, Episode 381, produced by Fred Diamond. https://www.salesgamechangerspodcast.com/mission/.

Hoebel, Tanya. "How These Leaders Discovered Their 'Why' After Conquering Chronic Illness and How It Applies to Sales." July 6, 2021, on *Sales Game Changers Podcast*, Episode 381, produced by Fred Diamond. https://www.salesgamechangerspodcast.com/mission/.

Ganong, Stephanie. 2020. "Lyme and Alcohol: Why I Don't Drink with Lyme Disease." Natural Paleo Family. https://www.naturalpaleofamily.com/dont-drink-with-lyme-disease/.

Health and Human Services. 2020. "TBDWG April 27, 2020 - Written Public Comment." https://www.hhs.gov/ash/advisory-committees/tickbornedisease/meetings/2020-4-27/written-public-comment/index.html.

Horowitz, Richard, MD. 2017. "Response to NY Times Article on 'Ethics' of Lyme Treatment." LymeDisease.org. https://www.lymedisease.org/response-ny-times-ethics-lyme-treatment/.

Houlis, A. 2022. "Alcohol and Inflammation." Alcohol Rehab Help. https://alcoholrehabhelp.org/addiction/inflammation.

Jagyasi, Prem, n.d. "Must Have Foods to Avoid Lyme Disease." Global Health Care. https://drprem.com/globalhealthcare/must-foods-avoid-lyme-disease.

Kenton, Will. 2021. "Regulatory Capture." Investopedia. https://www.investopedia.com/terms/r/regulatory-capture.asp.

Kirk, Gregg. 2017. "The Six Stages to Chronic Lyme Healing." The Gratitude Curve. https://greggkirk.com/the-gratitude-curve/.

Kirk, Gregg. "How These Leaders Discovered Their 'Why' After Conquering Chronic Illness and How It Applies to Sales." July 6, 2021, on *Sales Game Changers Podcast*, Episode 381, produced by Fred Diamond. https://www.salesgamechangerspodcast.com/mission/.

Lyme Warrior. n.d. "Heavy Metal & Lyme Disease." Accessed May 2022. https://lymewarrior.us/heavy-metals-lyme-disease.

Maderis, Todd. 2022. "Neurological Lyme Disease." Last updated February 6, 2022. https://drtoddmaderis.com/neurological-lyme-disease.

National Institute of Allergy and Infectious Diseases. 2022. "Lyme Disease Co-Infection." Last modified June 2022. https://www.niaid.nih.gov/diseases-conditions/lyme-disease-co-infection.

Nelson, T. J. "How TJ Nelson Excels at Sales While Battling Chronic Lyme Disease." September 23, 2021, on *Sales Game Changers Podcast*, Episode 410, produced by Fred Diamond. https://www.salesgamechangerspodcast.com/tjnelson/.

Sinusoid, Darya. 2021. "What Is Biohacking?—A Beginner's Guide." Shortform. https://www.shortform.com/blog/what-is-biohacking/.

Strasheim, Connie. 2016. *New Paradigms in Lyme Disease Treatment*. South Lake Tahoe, CA: BioMed Publishing Group.

Syritsyna, Olga, MD. 2022. "What's the Difference Between Neurologic Lyme Disease and MS?" Stonybrook University Hospital website. https://www.stonybrookmedicine.edu/patientcare/askexpert/neurologicallymediseaseandms.

Tired of Lyme. 2021. "Full Moons and Lyme Disease." https://www.tiredoflyme.com/full-moons-and-lyme-disease.html.

Wikipedia. 2022. "Chronic Lyme Disease." Last modified May 18, 2022, 00:28. https://en.wikipedia.org/wiki/Chronic_Lyme_disease.

APPENDIX A
Fifteen Books About Lyme I Recommend

Since I read over thirty books on Lyme and related topics, I'd like to suggest some you may want to get.

I put them into three categories:

1. **Lyme and Healing Overview**: These books provide a history of the disease and related coinfections, why and how it happens, its effects, and, most importantly, ways to treat it. Most of these were written by Lyme-literate medical professionals.
2. **Personal Stories**: There are a few memoirs of people's discovery of and battle with Lyme out there. In addition, a couple of celebrities have documented their history of having Lyme. One notable book was written by Yolanda Hadid of Housewives of Beverly Hills fame.
3. **Self-Care**: And there are some excellent books that cover how to treat depression, anxiety, and other related results of having Lyme disease.

The books below are available anywhere fine books are sold. I cannot vouch for the efficacy of what each author suggests, but the information was compelling.

Lyme and Healing Overview

Recovery from Lyme Disease: The Integrative Medicine Guide to Diagnosing and Treating Tick-Borne Illness, (2021), Dr. Daniel Kinderlehrer. I found this book to be very engaging, in-depth, and instructive. He delves deep into treatment, care, and strategies for success. Since it was just published in 2021, it's the most current book in this category.

How Can I Get Better? An Action Plan for Treating Resistant Lyme & Chronic Disease, (2017), Dr. Richard Horowitz. His first book on the topic, *Why Can't I Get Better?: Solving the Mystery of Lyme and Chronic Disease*, was published in 2015. It was the first book I read on Lyme, and it blew my mind. I couldn't believe how complicated treating Lyme could be. I then discovered he published *How Can I Get Better?* in 2017 and read that through. Horowitz is one of the most prominent Lyme-literate medical doctors and is frequently referenced in other books on the topic. The book is comprehensive in its coverage of Lyme and coinfections, and many treatment options are covered.

Toxic: Heal Your Body from Mold Toxicity, Lyme Disease, Multiple Chemical Sensitivities, and Chronic Environmental Illness, (2018), Dr. Neil Nathan. Healing was not a word I spent a lot of time thinking about before this summer, but of course, it's one Lyme survivors are frequently obsessed with. Like the Horowitz book above, I first read Nathan's predecessor, *Healing is Possible: New Hope for Chronic Fatigue, Fibromyalgia, Persistent Pain, and Other Chronic Illnesses*, published in 2013. Nathan practiced holistic medicine for over four decades before writing this book. His approach is very caring and sensitive.

Healing Lyme: Natural Healing of Lyme Borreliosis and the Coinfections Chlamydia and Spotted Fever Rickettsiosis, 2nd Edition, (2015), Stephen Buhner. If you suffer from Lyme, you probably are familiar with the herbal protocols available, and Buhner's is one of the most popular ones. Having treated tens of thousands of people, he has completed exhaustive work on this insidious disease and is one of the world's foremost experts on using herbals to treat Lyme and coinfections.

Insights into Lyme Disease Treatment: 13 Lyme-Literate Health Care Practitioners Share Their Healing Strategies, (2009), Connie Strasheim. Although she's written a few more books on Lyme since this one, I really enjoyed her approach here. She asked thirteen Lyme medical professionals to answer some basic questions about Lyme disease and to offer advice on treating mind, body, and spirit. Although it's over a decade since it was published, I found this book to be an excellent introduction to what the healing journey may look like and how to start building a treatment plan.

Autoimmune Illness and Lyme Disease Recovery Guide: Mending the Body, Mind, and Spirit, (2015), Katina Makris. The mind-body-spirit connection is critical for healing. Although many of the books above acknowledge that you need to address earlier life and childhood traumas you might have encountered before your body is ready to recover, this book goes deep into practice. I was especially impressed by the section on the seven chakras and how each plays a specific role in healing from Lyme.

Chronic: The Hidden Cause of the Autoimmune Pandemic and How to Get Healthy Again, (2021), Dr. Steven Phillips and Dana Parish. This was one of the first books I read, and it's a great place to get started understanding the epidemic that is chronic Lyme. It was one of the first books that helped me understand how much of a disconnect there is between what chronic Lyme patients suffer from and how the conventional medical community practices.

Lyme Brain: The Impact of Lyme Disease on Your Brain, and How to Reclaim Your Smarts, (2016), Dr. Nicola McFadzean Ducharme, ND. The title of the book caught my eye. My partner had sometimes complained about brain fog and had trouble concentrating. I was hoping to find some answers in this book.

Personal Stories

The Lady's Handbook for Her Mysterious Illness: A Memoir, (2021), Sarah Ramey. This book answered so many questions for me, as a male, and impacted me the deepest. I highly recommend it to any male partner who has questions about what his female partner's going through. I also recommend it to women with chronic Lyme who wonder why they go through what they go through to figure out how to solve their health challenges. Ramey bravely expounds on her journey, mistakes, and outcome. It's piercingly honest with a lot of tangents. If you love someone with Lyme, be it a partner, child, or other relative, your heart might get broken as you make it through this book.

The Gratitude Curve: Using the Lessons of Chronic Illness to Reach Personal Empowerment, (2018), Gregg Kirk. Like Sarah Ramey's book above, author Gregg Kirk goes very deep into his medical, physical, and spiritual journey to solve his health issues. I was so inspired by Kirk's story that I featured him on one of my *Sales Game Changers Podcast* episodes to talk about how he discovered his life's mission after accepting that he had Lyme disease.

Dear Lyme Disease: Transforming Your Pain into Purpose, (2020), Wendi Lindenmuth. Wendi shares her healing journey with Lyme disease and guides you through fourteen weeks of practical, alternative healing tools to help you heal. You will learn how to accept your "new normal," find hope, and transform your pain into purpose. (Note that Wendi helped me formulate the plan for my book.)

Lymebook: A Journey to Becoming One Day Better, (2021), J. P. Davitt. The author was a high-performing athlete and financial services professional before contracting Lyme. He shares his journey and documents in detail what he discovered along the way from other Lyme survivors and the medical community. Like Gregg Kirk, J. P.'s mission also became helping Lyme survivors with his Lymefriends community.

Self-Care

How to Heal Yourself from Depression When No One Else Can: A Self-Guided Program to Stop Feeling Like Sh*t, (2021), Amy Scher. The very first book I purchased when I began this endeavor was Amy's similarly titled book on healing from anxiety. Amy's a Lyme survivor and has written a half-dozen books on how to blossom even though you have the disease. Once I started reading these books, I noticed that many Lyme survivors were also dealing with devastating depression, stress, and anxiety. Amy suggests many practices you can take to handle depression to continue your healing journey.

Self-Love Workbook for Women: Release Self-Doubt, Build Self-Compassion, and Embrace Who You Are, (2020), Megan Logan. Having Lyme can affect your image, confidence, and psyche in ways you cannot even imagine. Many survivors remember their high levels of energy and performance before the disease took hold and look back on what's transpired forlornly. That doesn't have to happen. In this book, the author has created numerous exercises to help you build back your confidence and enjoy your life again.

The Emotion Code: How to Release Your Trapped Emotions for Abundant Health, Love, and Happiness (Updated and Expanded Edition), (2019), Dr. Bradley Nelson. While not specifically about recovering from Lyme, this book explores how releasing trapped emotions throughout your body can help accelerate healing. It's a fascinating process.

Acknowledgments

If you had told me that the first book I would ever write would be about Lyme disease, I would have said probably not. However, none of this would have been possible without some amazing people. Some I've known for decades, and some I met when I realized I needed to learn more about Lyme disease and how it affects families.

None of this would have been possible without my amazing editor Wendi Lindenmuth. Her book, *Dear Lyme Disease: Transforming Your Pain into Purpose*, was one of the first Lyme books I read, and I was honored to have her edit my manuscript and make it coherent. I am so fortunate to have come across her book.

I am lucky to have two amazing parents, Joan and Herbert Diamond, who have shown me what a loving couple can be for each other. Over sixty years married and still in love. Until death do they part.

Thank you to my three kids, I have one of each, Steven, Andi, and Abby, for listening to me as I processed what I was learning and for bringing me joy every day.

I am grateful for my sister Bonnie, brother-in-law Doug, and my niece Allison and nephew David.

At the beginning of this process, I knew one person with Lyme disease. However, throughout the writing of this book, I met so many amazing people who have helped me understand the challenges Lyme survivors face and the possibilities they have in their lives once they accept that they have Lyme. I'm grateful to J. P. Davitt, Tanya Hoebel, Bill Syrjala, Shannon Pinkston, and the many others who helped me understand what they go through every day.

Thanks to Dorothy Leland at LymeDisease.org for posting blogs I've written for partners and family members of Lyme survivors.

Thanks to Gregg Kirk for his help on the chapter on healing. His book, *The Gratitude Curve*, was one of the first I'd read as well.

Gina Stracuzzi is an amazing colleague at the Institute for Excellence in Sales. She has done a spectacular job growing our Women in Sales program, which has helped hundreds of women in sales take their lives and careers to the next level. Thank you for what you do for women in the workforce.

Thanks to the team at Eaton Press for publishing my book.

And for one person I'll always love, hopefully this book will help many Lyme survivors find peace, support, love, and hope.

About the Author

Fred Diamond is the cofounder of the Institute for Excellence in Sales and the host and producer of the award-winning *Sales Game Changers Podcast*. He is the author of *Insights for Sales Game Changers*.

His favorite saying is the Einstein quote, "Only a life lived in the service to others is a life worth living."

He is a graduate of Emory University and has an MBA from San Jose State University. He lives in Fairfax, Virginia.

He wishes that more people were aware of the devastation Lyme disease and other tick-borne illnesses can cause.

A portion of the profits from this book will be distributed to various Lyme disease charities.

For more information, visit www.lovehopelyme.com.

Epilogue

I despise cliches such as "Everything happens for a reason" or "When one door closes, another opens."

Same with "If you love something, set it free. If it comes back, it's yours. If not, it wasn't meant to be."

I've heard that over 75 percent of committed relationships end when one of the partners has a chronic illness, such as Lyme disease.

That's unfortunate. It's sad.

Recovering from chronic illness, specifically Lyme disease, is challenging and can become an all-consuming chore for the survivor. Sometimes, the overwhelming nature of the disease can overtake the relationship, as it did in this one.

But remember that love will never die, and there is always hope.

Made in the USA
Middletown, DE
22 February 2023